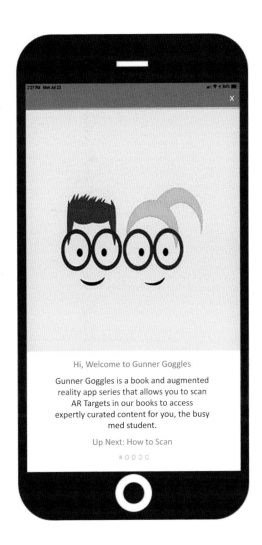

GUNNER GOGGLES

Neurology

HONORS SHELF REVIEW

EDITORS:

Hao-Hua Wu, MD
Resident, Department of Orthopaedic Surgery
University of California–San Francisco
San Francisco, California

Leo Wang, MS, PhD
Perelman School of Medicine
University of Pennsylvania
Philadelphia, Pennsylvania

FACULTY EDITOR:
Chuang-Kuo Wu, MD, PhD
University of California Irvine School of Medicine
Irvine, California

ELSEVIER

ELSEVIER

1600 John F. Kennedy Blvd.
Ste 1800
Philadelphia, PA 19103-2899

GUNNER GOGGLES NEUROLOGY, HONORS SHELF REVIEW   ISBN: 978-0-323-51036-3

Library of Congress Cataloging-in-Publication Data
Names: Wu, Hao-Hua, editor. | Wang, Leo, editor. | Wu, Chuang-Kuo, editor.
Title: Gunner goggles neurology : honors shelf review / editors, Hao-Hua Wu, Leo Wang ; faculty editor, Chuang-Kuo Wu.
Description: Philadelphia, PA : Elsevier, [2019] | Includes bibliographical references.
Identifiers: LCCN 2017040716 | ISBN 9780323510363 (pbk. : alk. paper)
Subjects: | MESH: Nervous System Diseases | Test Taking Skills | User-Computer Interface | Study Guide
Classification: LCC BF176 | NLM WL 18.2 | DDC 150.28/7--dc23 LC record available at https://lccn.loc.gov/2017040716

Executive Content Strategist: Jim Merritt
Content Development Manager: Lucia Gunzel
Publishing Services Manager: Patricia Tannian
Senior Project Manager: Cindy Thoms
Senior Book Designer: Maggie Reid

  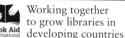

Working together
to grow libraries in
developing countries

www.elsevier.com • www.bookaid.org

Printed in China

Last digit is the print number: 9 8 7 6 5 4 3 2 1

Gunner Goggles Honors Shelf Review Series

Gunner Goggles Family Medicine 978-0-323-51034-9

Gunner Goggles Medicine 978-0-323-51035-6

Gunner Goggles Neurology 978-0-323-51036-3

Gunner Goggles Obstetrics and Gynecology 978-0-323-51037-0

Gunner Goggles Pediatrics 978-0-323-51038-7

Gunner Goggles Psychiatry 978-0-323-51039-4

Gunner Goggles Surgery 978-0-323-51040-0

Contributors

SECTION EDITOR

Michael Baer, MD
Resident, Department of Neurology, University of Pennsylvania, Philadelphia, Pennsylvania
Degenerative and Global Cerebral Dysfunction Disorders
Neuromuscular Disorders, Movement Disorders

CONTRIBUTING AUTHORS

Catherine Blebea, BS
Perelman School of Medicine, University of Pennsylvania, Philadelphia, Pennsylvania
Metabolic Disorders on the Neurology Shelf

George Hung, BS
Perelman School of Medicine, University of Pennsylvania, Philadelphia, Pennsylvania
Neoplasms of the Nervous System
Disorders of the Cranial Nerves and Peripheral Nervous System

Diana Kim, MD
Resident Physician, Department of Ophthalmology, University of Pennsylvania,
Philadelphia, Pennsylvania
Disorders of the Special Senses

Acknowledgments

"If I have seen further than others, it is by standing upon the shoulders of giants."
–Isaac Newton

We would like to thank the many exceptional innovators who helped transform our vision of *Gunner Goggles Neurology* into reality.

To our editorial team at Elsevier, thank you for your unrelenting support throughout the publication process. Jim Merritt believed in *Gunner Goggles* from day one and used his experience as an executive content strategist to point us in the right direction with respect to book proposal, product pitch, and manuscript development. Margaret Nelson and Lucia Gunzel expertly guided us through manuscript submission and revision, no easy feat with two first-time authors. Maggie Reid collaborated with us closely to create the layout design and color schemes. Cindy Thoms and the copy editing team made sure our written content adhered to a high professional standard.

To the editors, authors, and student reviewers of *Gunner Goggles Neurology*, thank you for your scholarship and unwavering enthusiasm. Dr. Chuang-Kuo Wu took time out of his busy clinical practice to meticulously edit each chapter, and he provided numerous invaluable insights on how we could improve quality and accuracy. A number of outstanding residents and medical students contributed to the content of this textbook and provided us feedback on high-yield topics for the NBME Clinical Neurology Subject Exam, notably Dr. Michael Baer, Dr. Diana Kim, George Hung, and Catherine Blebea.

To our augmented reality (AR) team, thank you for your creativity and dedication during the development of the *Gunner Goggles* AR application. Nadir Bilici, Brian Mayo, Vlad Obsekov, Clare Teng, and Yinka Orafidiya helped us develop and test the initial *Gunner Goggles* AR prototype. Tammy Bui designed the *Gunner Goggles* logo and AR app icon.

We would also like to thank the Wharton Innovation Fund for awarding us seed money to help pursue development of *Gunner Goggles* AR.

You all continue to inspire us, and we are incredibly grateful and deeply appreciative for your support.

–Hao-Hua and Leo

Contents

Introduction

Hao-Hua Wu and Leo Wang

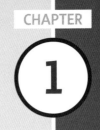

I. Gunner's Guide to a Better Test Score

Curious why certain classmates perform well on every exam? Frustrated by how few of these "gunner" peers share study secrets?

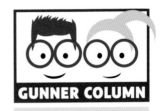

At *Gunner Goggles* (GG), our goal is to reveal and demystify. By integrating *augmented reality* (AR) into this review book, we reveal how some of the best students approach topics, conceptualize complex disease, and allocate study time efficiently. By organizing each topic according to the National Board of Medical Examiners (NBME) format, we demystify exam content and the types of questions one can expect on test day.

Of the tests medical students strive to conquer, shelf exams boast the highest ratio of importance to quality of study resources. For instance, performance on shelf exams typically informs final clerkship grades, which are the most important criteria on the medical school transcript for residency application. Yet, there is no single authoritative study resource for the shelf across all disciplines. Most importantly, no current book specifically targets shelf exam prep, so students must rely on miscellaneous resources and anecdotal advice to get the job done.

In light of this void in authoritative test prep, we have created the *GG* series to provide you with the most effective shelf exam testing resource. *GG* stands out for three important reasons:

First, readers have the opportunity to enhance understanding of important shelf topics by using the AR features on each page. With an iPhone or iPad, users can download the *Gunner Goggles* AR iOS app and use it to turn book figures into three-dimensional (3D) images, access high-yield videos and view pertinent digital media. More on how AR technology works can be found in the next section.

Second, *GG* provides a plethora of tips on how to manage time efficiently when studying for the shelf. Mnemonics and strategies for how to approach difficult concepts can be found in the blue "Gunner Column" to the right or left of each page. We also tell you how to *think* about these concepts so that medicine never feels like a laundry list of items you simply have to memorize.

Third, this review book is written and organized optimally for shelf exam test prep. Each chapter is organized according to the NBME Shelf Exam and USMLE course content outlines. In addition, a concise summary of how topics are tested prefaces each chapter.

As experts on the shelf exam, we understand how difficult it is to carve out time to study while juggling clinical responsibilities during your clerkship rotation. We also know that each student's learning curve is different based on timing of the rotation (first block vs. last block), year in medical school (MS3 vs. MD/PhD returning after graduate school), and future career interests (e.g., an aspiring orthopedic surgeon learning about obstetrics and gynecology). However, we believe that any student can perform well on the shelf exam with the right strategy and study resources.

We created this book anticipating the needs of all types of students and hope that *Gunner Goggles* will be the most comprehensive, authoritative shelf exam review book that you ever use. We are confident that *Gunner Goggles* will enable you to achieve your test performance goals and stick it to your "gunner" classmates, whose advice, or lack thereof, you won't be needing after all.

II. Augmented Reality: A New Paradigm for Shelf Exam Test Prep

Think of AR as your best friend.

To use it, download the free *Gunner Goggles Neurology* application on your iPad or iPhone and create your own optional profile. Now with the *application* open, point your smart mobile camera at this page.

Notice how on your camera, there are now links you can click on, 3D figures you can rotate, and a video you can watch. You have just unlocked the AR features for this page!

Take a moment to play around with these AR features on your smart mobile device. The way this works is that anytime you see the "Gunner Goggles" icon **gg** in the blue Gunner Column to the right or left, there is an AR feature accompanying the text with which you have the opportunity to interact.

Still not convinced? Here are three reasons why AR is your ideal study companion.

gg AR

Gunner Goggles Introduction Video

gg AR

Gunner Goggles Contact

Presentation

AR breaks the boundaries of how information can be presented in this textbook.

Traditionally, if you wanted to learn about a disease in a review book, you would be expected to read and memorize a block of text similar to the following:

"Huntington disease (HD) is a GABAergic neurodegenerative disorder that is caused by an autosomal dominant mutation leading to CAG repeats on chromosome 4. Patients typically present in the fourth and fifth decade of life with chorea, memory loss, caudate atrophy on neuroimaging and motor impairment, depending on the variant. Although there is no cure for HD, the movement disorders associated with the disease, such as chorea, can be treated with drugs like tetrabenazine and reserpine to decrease dopamine release."

Having read (or most likely glazed) through that previous paragraph, do you feel comfortable enough to answer questions about the genetics, presentation, and treatment of HD right now? A week from now? Three weeks from now when you have to take your shelf exam?

Here's where AR comes in. Use your *GG* app to check out how we're able to present HD in different, memorable ways.

For visual learners, here's a video of an effective HD mnemonic →

AR
Huntington Disease Mnemonic

If you are an audio learner, here's a link to key points about HD for the shelf →

AR
Huntington Disease Podcast

Forgot your neuroanatomy? Here's where the caudate is →

AR
The caudate nucleus is part of the basal ganglia

What's the difference between chorea, athetosis, and ballismus again? Chorea looks like this →

AR
Chorea patient example

Now write a one-line description of HD in your own words in the margins of this page for future reference. It's much easier with AR, right? Like we said, your best friend.

Evaluation

The GG Neurology app has the potential to exponentially enhance how you can evaluate your own understanding of the material. Although not available with the first edition, we are in the process of developing a personalized question bank as well as a flashcards feature. Our vision is to allow you to scan a topic on the page for immediate access to relevant practice questions and flashcards. In future versions, you will also be able to create your own flashcard deck and track your mastery.

In addition the GG app can keep track of the AR Targets scanned and the Learning links viewed. These links are saved to a Link Library which you can view at any time.

You can also like or dislike a Learning Link with an opportunity to provide us feedback for better resources available.

As development of the GG Neurology app is an ongoing process, we encourage and welcome your feedback. If you like the idea of having a personalized question bank and flashcard feature or have an idea for how we can improve the GG app to better serve your studying needs, please provide us feedback through an in-app message. You can also email us at GunnerGoggles@gmail.com.

Community Engagement

Studying for the shelf can be isolating. Our vision is to develop a feature in the GG Neurology that would allow you to connect with chapter authors and fellow readers. We are in the process of developing a medium in which shelf-related inquiries can be discussed among authors and readers through an optional short message system (SMS) feature.

99 AR
Gunner Goggles Forum

Given that the community engagement feature is in development and unavailable for the first edition, we welcome your input on how we can connect you with the people who will enable your test day success.

To provide feedback, please scan the page and vote. You can also email us GunnerGoggles@gmail.com for any comments or suggestions.

Augmented Reality Frequently Asked Questions

"Since AR is integrated into *Gunner Goggles Neurology*, does this mean I have to pull out my iPad of iPhone for every page of the book?"

No, only if you need it. Some may use AR more than others, depending on background and level of comfort with neurology. For instance, you may already have a solid understanding of HD and need to read only the text as a refresher. On the other hand, if you are less comfortable with HD, the AR features are there just in case.

"Can't I just look up everything I don't know on my own? Why do I have to use the *Gunner Goggles* app?"

You can absolutely look things up on your own, but that takes time. And sometimes, you can't find the best reference or mnemonic. We have already gone through the trouble of identifying potential sources of confusion for you and found the perfect resources. In the *Gunner Goggles* app, we have compiled the slickest and most concise resources one can use to better understand a topic. Videos, audio files, and images are first vetted by subject experts for accuracy of content. They are then evaluated by students like yourself for utility of content to enhance test performance. Only resources with the most Gunner votes are embedded into each page.

"What if a link doesn't work or I want something on the page to change?"

Please tell us! Another advantage of AR is that we can immediately receive and implement your feedback. Just use the *Gunner Goggles* app to text us your concerns, and our tech support team will respond ASAP!

III. Study Smart: Mnemonics and Gunner Study Tips

Even with incredible AR features at your disposal, you won't be able to optimize exam performance unless you know how to study. Below are the four most important things one can do to study for the shelf under the time restraints imposed by clerkships.

Understand the Organizing Principle

The easiest way to both save time and perform well on the shelf is to understand how a specific disease or concept fits into the big picture. For instance, knowing the mechanism, diagnostic criteria, and treatment plan for HD will likely lead to only one correct answer on the test. However, understanding that HD exists on a spectrum of neurodegenerative disorders presenting with memory loss can enhance your ability to answer any question in which patient recall is an issue. Thus, when you read about HD, be sure to differentiate it from dementia, Alzheimer disease, and amnesia, which are all disorders that can lead to memory impairment. Forcing yourself to make these connections and compare diseases among themselves is a relatively quick mental exercise that can greatly deepen your understanding of the material.

Create Effective Mnemonics

If you have photographic memory, skip this section. For the rest of us mere mortals, the organizing principles (OPs) of what constitutes a Gunner mnemonic are outlined next.

Mnemonics are important when

1. You have to learn a lot of material.
2. You want to teach something to your colleagues during morning rounds. Attendings and residents are always impressed when they can learn something from a medical student.

3. You want to remember something 15 years from now when you are working the 30th hour of a busy call day. OPs for mnemonics are as follows:
    1. Use the spelling of a name to your benefit (Spell)
       Example:
        i. "8urk14tt" lymphoma (Burkitt lymphoma), "lep"thin" (leptin), "supraoptiuretic" nuclei (supraoptic nuclei that produces antidiuretic hormone)
        ii. Tenofovir is the only NRTI nucleoTide
        iii. We"C"ener granulomatosis (GPA) for C-ANCA and Cyclophosphamide treatment

    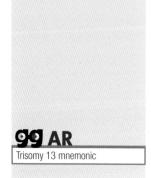
    Trisomy 13 mnemonic

    2. Create an acronym that contains distinguishing syllables or letters of names (Distinguish)
       Example:
        i. Chronic Alcoholics Steal PhenPhen and Nevar Rifuse Grisee Carbs (<u>Chronic alcohol</u> abuse + <u>St.</u> John's wort + <u>pheny</u>toin + <u>pheno</u>barb + <u>nevari</u>pine + <u>rif</u>ampin + <u>grise</u>ofulvin + <u>carb</u>amazepine)
            • Reinforce mnemonic by spelling name of item to be memorized accordingly
                • e.g. "Refus"ampin, "Never"apine, "Greasy" ofulvin, "Carb"amazepine, etc.
                • This ties mnemonic OP 1 with mnemonic OP 2
    3. Drawings help (Draw)
       Example: Trisomy 13 looks like polydactyly + cleft lip when the number 13 is rotated 90 degrees clockwise (the horizontal 1 is the extra digit, and the cleft of the horizontal 3 is the cleft lip)
    4. Counting the letters of a word (Count)
       Example: Patau syndrome = 13 letters = Trisomy 13
    5. Arrange acronym in alphabetical order (Arrange)
       Example: ABCDEF for diphtheria (ADP ribosylation, beta prophage, Corynebacterium diphtheriae, elongation factor 2)
       Examples of instructors who practice this concept well are Dr. John Barone of Kaplan and Dr. Husain Sattar of Pathoma.
       On the flip side, here are examples of poor mnemonics (although you may remember them now given how they were highlighted in this text).
    i. Blind as a bat, mad as a hatter, red as a beet, hot as Hades, dry as a bone, the bowel and bladder lose their tone, and the heart runs alone = poor mnemonic for anticholinergic syndrome
        • This mnemonic forces you to memorize extra and extraneous things (like bat, beet, hare, and desert) that have nothing to do with anticholinergic syndrome.
    ii. WWHHHHIMP (withdrawal + wernicke + hypertensive crisis + hypoxia + hypoglycemia + hypoperfusion +

intracranial bleed + meningitis/encephalopathy + poisoning) = poor mnemonic for causes of delirium
- Wait, how many *H*s does this mnemonic have again?

A good rule of thumb: if you can still remember a mnemonic under a high-pressure situation (attending pimps you) or after a 7-day period, then you have a winner.

Ultimately, the best mnemonics are the ones you invent and apply repeatedly, so use these mnemonic principles to give yourself a solid head start.

Devise a Study Schedule and Stick to It

The third most important piece of advice for the shelf is to create a study schedule at the beginning of the rotation and follow it. Rotations are draining, and oftentimes you may find yourself coming home after a 12-hour shift not wanting to study. However, if you are mentally committed to following a schedule, you will find creative ways to get studying done. For example, some students wake up an hour early to read before pre-rounds. Other students fit study material into their white coat and read during downtime.

Distinguish Rotation-Knowledge From Shelf-Knowledge

Most things you learn on rotation do not apply to the shelf exam and vice versa. For example, you may be able to impress your neurology attending by committing the National Institutes of Health (NIH) Stroke Scale to memory. However, with only 150 minutes to answer 100 lengthy questions on the shelf, diagnostic scores like that have no real utility.

Thus, be able to compartmentalize. Knowing exactly what is needed for clinics and what is expected on the shelf can save you a lot of precious study time.

IV. Intro to the National Board of Medical Examiners Clinical Neurology Shelf

NBME Shelf Exam Website

The Clinical Neurology NBME Shelf Exam is a 110-question computerized exam administered over a recommended course of 2 hours and 45 minutes, typically at the conclusion of one's neurology clerkship rotation. The test questions come from either retired Step 2 Clinical Knowledge (CK) questions or are written by a committee of faculty across the country. Thus it is important to master shelf exam–style questions to set yourself up nicely for Step 2 CK.

Unlike Step 1, shelf exam questions focus almost exclusively on disease processes rather than normal processes. That being said, the most high-yield normal process to know for the neurology shelf is normal aging because question writers are known to present you a question stem of normal aging phenomena and try to trick you with pathologic answer choices.

According to the NBME, the exams are curved to a mean of 70, with a standard deviation of 8. The curve does not take into account timing of rotation. For instance, students who take the exam during their first block will be held to the same statistical standard as students who take the exam during their fourth clerkship block. However, the NBME does release "quarterly norm information" to medical schools to make clerkship directors aware of the relationship between exam score and rotation timing. Importantly, as of now, shelf exam scores are sent to the school directly; students cannot request their shelf exam score independent of their school.

Although different neurology clerkships have different standards for determining grades, in general, each program has its own internally generated shelf exam cutoff score one needs to achieve to be eligible for the highest clerkship grade (e.g., Honors). If this is the case, confirm the cutoff score with your clerkship director so that you have a reasonable performance goal to shoot for.

Students are expected to master content organized into these following categories:

99 AR

Clinical Neurology Outline

TABLE 1.1 Clinical Neurology Subject Examination Content Outline

System		
General Principles, Including Normal Age-Related Findings and Care of the Well Patient	1%–5%	
Behavioral Health	3%–7%	
Nervous System & Special Senses	60%–65%	
Infectious, immunologic, and inflammatory disorders		
Neoplasms (cerebral, spinal, and peripheral)		
Cerebrovascular disease		
Disorders related to the spine, spinal cord, and spinal nerve roots		
Cranial and peripheral nerve disorders		
Neurologic pain syndromes		
Degenerative disorders/amnestic syndromes		
Global cerebral dysfunction		
Neuromuscular disorders		
Movement disorders		
Paroxysmal disorders		
Sleep disorders		
Traumatic and mechanical disorders and disorders of increased intracranial pressure		

TABLE 1.1 Clinical Neurology Subject Examination Content Outline—cont'd

System	
Congenital disorders	
Adverse effects of drugs on the nervous system	
Disorders of the eye and ear	
Musculoskeletal System	10%–15%
Other Systems, Including Multisystem Processes & Disorders	15%–20%
Social Sciences, Including Death and Dying and Palliative Care	1%–5%

Adapted from the National Board of Medical Examiners website. http://www.nbme.org/Schools/Subject-Exams/Subjects /clinicalsci_neur.html

Currently, the NBME Clinical Neurology Content Outline breaks down question types into three categories

- Applying Foundational Science Concepts (10%-15%)
- Diagnosis: Knowledge Pertaining to History, Exam, Diagnostic Studies, & Patient Outcomes (55%-60%)
- Health Maintenance, Pharmacotherapy, Intervention & Management (25%-30%)

However, devising a study plan from these three categories can be confusing. "Applying Foundational Science Concepts," for instance, is vague and difficult to prepare for. Instead, many students prefer to study according to Physician Tasks provided in older content outlines. Since every subject exam question asks about one of four things – 1) protocol for promoting health maintenance (Prophylaxis [PPx]), 2) the mechanism of disease (MoD), 3) steps to establishing a diagnosis (Dx), and 4) steps of disease management (Tx/Mgmt) – we recommend studying according to Physician Tasks from the 2016 Content Outline.

Physician Tasks (from 2016 Content Outline)

Promoting Health and Health Maintenance	5%–10%
Understanding Mechanisms of Disease	15%–20%
Establishing a Diagnosis	50%–65%
Applying Principles of Management	15%–20%

In addition, the NBME breaks down questions by Site of Care,

- Ambulatory (60%-65%)
- Emergency Department (25%-30%)
- Inpatient (5%-15%)

And by Patient Age:

- Birth to 17 (10%-15%)
- 18 to 65 (55%-65%)
- 66 and older (20%-25%)

Our recommendation is to not worry about site of care or age; instead, focus on studying content related to Physician Tasks.

Gunner Goggles Neurology presents material to reflect how the NBME structures its shelf exams. Each chapter that follows falls into the main testable categories of General Principles (Chapter 2), Mental Disorders (Chapter 3), Diseases of the Nervous System and Special Senses (Chapters 4–16), and Other Organ Systems (Chapters 17–18). The "Musculoskeletal System" portion of the exam will be covered in Chapter 10. Each disease is presented in a "PPx, MoD, Dx, and Tx/Mgmt" format, which represents the four physician tasks they can test you on. Because establishing a diagnosis is weighted especially heavily (50%–65%), the "Buzz Words" category shows readers how to quickly identify the disease process from just a few key words. The "Clinical Presentation" section serves to more thoroughly describe the disease. However, it is important to note that Buzz Words are sufficient in correctly identifying the corresponding disease on the shelf. The detail provided in the Clinical Presentation section is meant only to augment your understanding, particularly if it is your first pass and you are unfamiliar with the material. However, by the end of studying, the focus should primarily be on Buzz Words.

Finally, here are four things to keep in mind when studying for the shelf.

1. If pressed for time, practice identifying disease processes only through "Buzz Words." For instance, a patient with atrophy of the caudate nucleus and progressive memory loss should immediately evoke HD. Patients with sclerosing cholangitis on the shelf exam always have underlying ulcerative colitis.
2. Many questions given in the neurology shelf can double count for another exam topic. Thus, watch out for cases that present like a neurologic disease but are treated by other specialties (i.e., a patient presenting with memory loss who is primarily afflicted with a psychiatric disorder).
3. Make sure to begin doing questions early (e.g., 10 questions a day starting from day 1). Ideally you should make a second pass of the most high-yield questions.
4. For each question, write a one-line take-home point in an Excel spreadsheet. This makes for quick and easy review in the days leading up to the exam.

If any questions arise while studying, use the *Gunner Goggles* app to access the AR features embedded on each page. Good luck and happy hunting.

—The *Gunner Goggles* Team

General Principles for the Neurology Shelf Exam

Hao-Hua Wu, Leo Wang, and Chuang-Kuo Wu

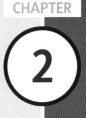
As a student, studying "General Principles" for the neurology shelf exam means learning what is normal. One requires an understanding of normal processes (e.g., autonomic nervous system [ANS], cranial nerves) to understand disease pathology from those areas. Thus, although questions pertaining specifically to general principles comprise only 1%–5% of the test (more likely closer to 1%), you will need the knowledge to stand a better chance at answering the other 95%–99% of questions. That being said, if you have a strong background in neuroscience, please skip directly to the Gunner Practice section.

This chapter focuses on the nervous system (central nervous system [CNS] and peripheral nervous system [PNS]), as well as miscellaneous high-yield general principle topics. Basic science topics such as the structure of a neuron, types of neurotransmitters, and principles of action potentials are not covered, because they are more aligned with Step 1. Mastery of basic science topics is not essential, but for those of you who lack confidence on the most basic neurologic premises, peruse the links on this page's Gunner Column.

In general, use the figures provided to understand how the CNS and PNS are organized. This will enable you to feel more comfortable with neuroanatomic terms seen in shelf question stems.

Most importantly, be comfortable with the most commonly tested general principles, such as normal aging, which can be found under the third miscellaneous section.

Remember, unlike Step 1, the neurology shelf exam focuses primarily on disease processes. Thus it is unlikely to see a question that asks specifically about normal function. However, it is likely that knowledge of the normal function can lead to the right answer.

Finally, this chapter is meant to be referenced many times throughout your course of study. Do not be discouraged if you do not remember most of what you read during your first pass. Move on to other chapters, do questions, and flip back to this chapter as needed.

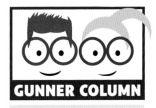

GUNNER COLUMN

Neuroscience review

Central Nervous System (Fig. 2.1)

The CNS is one half of the nervous system (the PNS being the other part of the equation). The CNS is composed of brain and spinal cord. For the shelf, be able to organize the structures by embryologic origin such that if you were to see a structure like "amygdala" on the test, you would know generally where it resides.

The "brain" portion of the CNS can be divided into three embryologic entities: forebrain (telencephalon, diencephalon), midbrain (mesencephalon), and hindbrain (metencephalon, myelencephalon). Do not memorize these categorizations; instead, memorize the fact that there are five different embryologic regions of the brain that all anatomic structures fall into.

After you have a good sense of what goes where (i.e., midbrain is in the middle brain region and connects diencephalon with metencephalon), you'll have a much easier time localizing the lesion.

Brain (Fig. 2.2)

A. Forebrain

The forebrain contains all brain structures except for the cerebellum and brain stem. It further subdivides into the telencephalon and diencephalon.

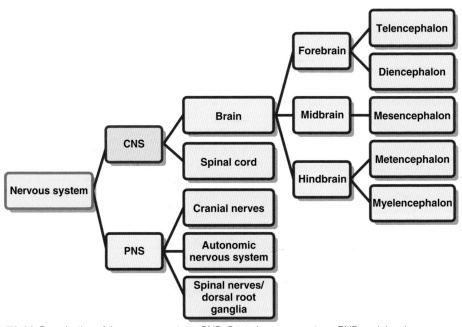

FIG. 2.1 Organization of the nervous system. *CNS*, Central nervous system; *PNS*, peripheral nervous system.

The telencephalon includes the cerebral cortex (i.e., frontal, parietal, temporal, occipital lobes), subcortical white matter, basal ganglia, and amygdala (Fig. 2.3). The diencephalon includes the thalamus and hypothalamus. Again, it is not necessary to memorize embryologic origin for the shelf (i.e., you will never get a question asking the embryologic origin of the basal ganglia). However, it is useful to understand the grouping of the structures, such as how the thalamus and hypothalamus are interconnected with the limbic system.

1. Frontal Lobe

Anatomic borders: Posteriorly separated from parietal lobe by central sulcus; inferiorly separated from temporal lobe by sylvian fissure

Significance: Contains Broca area (produces intelligible speech), primary motor cortex (sends motor commands to entire body), and prefrontal association cortex (controls planning behavior)

Notable disease manifestations: Broca aphasia, hemiparesis 2/2 stroke, disinhibition 2/2 frontotemporal dementia (FTD), primitive behaviors, abulia

Vascular supply: Anterior cerebral artery (ACA), middle cerebral artery (MCA)

2. Parietal Lobe (Fig. 2.4)

Anatomic borders: Anteriorly separated from frontal lobe by central sulcus; posteriorly separated from occipital lobe by parietooccipital sulcus in the medial aspect of the hemisphere; inferiorly separated from temporal

> **QUICK TIPS**
> Primary motor cortex = Precentral gyrus (frontal lobe). Primary somatosensory cortex = Postcentral gyrus (parietal lobe).

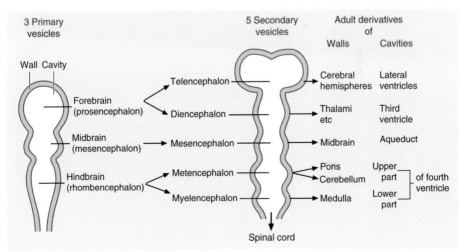

FIG. 2.2 Forebrain, midbrain, and hindbrain. (From Coady A. Cranial abnormalities. In: Coady A, Bower S, eds. *Twining's Textbook of Fetal Abnormalities*. 3rd ed. London: Elsevier Ltd; 2015.)

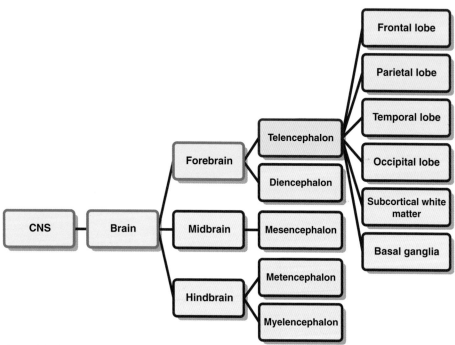

FIG. 2.3 Forebrain structures derived from the telencephalon. *CNS,* Central nervous system.

lobe by sylvian fissure; no clear landmark on the lateral aspect of hemisphere

Significance: Contains primary somatosensory cortex (receives body sensory input), posterior parietal association area (visual-motor perception), tertiary somatosensory cortex (stereognosis)

Notable disease manifestations: Numbness 2/2 stroke, hemineglect 2/2 stroke, Gerstmann syndrome, apraxia, anosognosia, extinction, hemineglect

Vascular supply: ACA, MCA

3. Temporal Lobe

Anatomic borders: Superiorly separated from frontal/parietal lobe by sylvian fissure

Significance: Contains Wernicke area (speech comprehension), primary auditory cortex (also known as [aka] Heschl gyri; hearing), hippocampus (memory), amygdala (emotions)

Notable disease manifestations: Wernicke aphasia, Alzheimer disease (hippocampal pathology), Klüver-Bucy syndrome (amygdala pathology)

Vascular supply: ACA, MCA

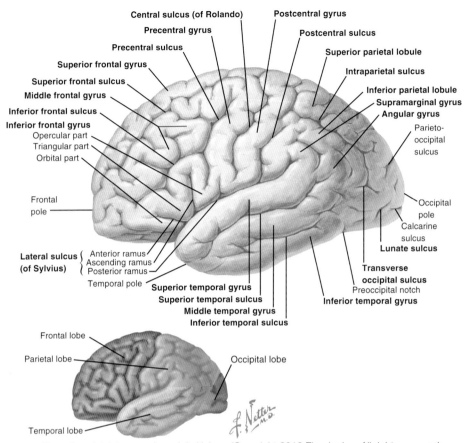

Central sulcus (of Rolando)
Precentral gyrus
Precentral sulcus
Superior frontal gyrus
Superior frontal sulcus
Middle frontal gyrus
Inferior frontal sulcus
Inferior frontal gyrus
Opercular part
Triangular part
Orbital part
Frontal pole
Lateral sulcus (of Sylvius) { Anterior ramus / Ascending ramus / Posterior ramus }
Temporal pole
Superior temporal gyrus
Superior temporal sulcus
Middle temporal gyrus
Inferior temporal sulcus

Postcentral gyrus
Postcentral sulcus
Superior parietal lobule
Intraparietal sulcus
Inferior parietal lobule
Supramarginal gyrus
Angular gyrus
Parieto-occipital sulcus
Occipital pole
Calcarine sulcus
Lunate sulcus
Transverse occipital sulcus
Preoccipital notch
Inferior temporal gyrus

Frontal lobe
Parietal lobe
Occipital lobe
Temporal lobe

FIG. 2.4 Frontal, parietal, temporal, occipital lobes. (Copyright 2016 Elsevier Inc. All rights reserved. http://www.netterimages.com.)

4. Occipital Lobe
Anatomic borders: Anteriorly and medially separated from parietal lobe by parietooccipital gyrus; no clear lateral demarcation
Significance: Contains primary visual cortex (vision)
Notable disease manifestations: Loss of central vision 2/2 stroke, achromatopsia, prosopagnosia, palinopsia
Vascular supply: Posterior cerebral artery (PCA)
5. Subcortical White Matter
Anatomic borders: Axons that carry signals among all the lobes and between the two hemispheres of the cerebral cortex, as well as from cerebral cortex to other neuroanatomic regions
Significance: Contains corpus callosum, internal capsule, external capsule

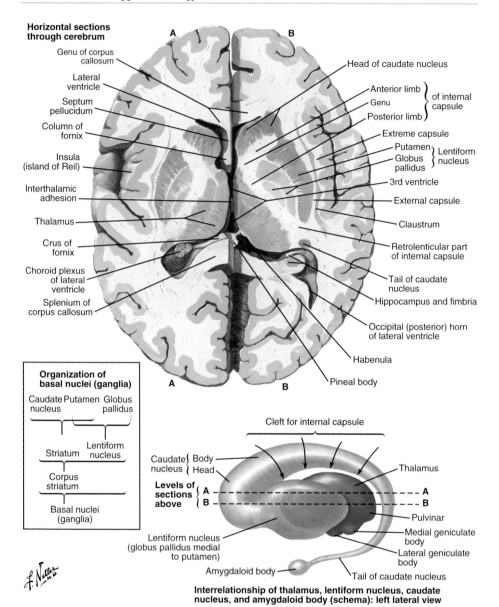

Horizontal sections through cerebrum

- Genu of corpus callosum
- Lateral ventricle
- Septum pellucidum
- Column of fornix
- Insula (island of Reil)
- Interthalamic adhesion
- Thalamus
- Crus of fornix
- Choroid plexus of lateral ventricle
- Splenium of corpus callosum

- Head of caudate nucleus
- Anterior limb ⎫
- Genu ⎬ of internal capsule
- Posterior limb ⎭
- Extreme capsule
- Putamen ⎫ Lentiform
- Globus pallidus ⎬ nucleus
- 3rd ventricle
- External capsule
- Claustrum
- Retrolenticular part of internal capsule
- Tail of caudate nucleus
- Hippocampus and fimbria
- Occipital (posterior) horn of lateral ventricle
- Habenula
- Pineal body

Organization of basal nuclei (ganglia)

Caudate nucleus — Putamen — Globus pallidus

Striatum / Lentiform nucleus

Corpus striatum

Basal nuclei (ganglia)

Cleft for internal capsule

- Caudate nucleus { Body / Head
- Levels of sections above { A / B
- Lentiform nucleus (globus pallidus medial to putamen)
- Amygdaloid body
- Thalamus
- Pulvinar
- Medial geniculate body
- Lateral geniculate body
- Tail of caudate nucleus

Interrelationship of thalamus, lentiform nucleus, caudate nucleus, and amygdaloid body (schema): left lateral view

FIG. 2.5 Anatomic location of the basal ganglia. (Copyright 2016 Elsevier Inc. All rights reserved. http://www.netterimages.com.)

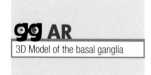

3D Model of the basal ganglia

Notable disease manifestations: Loss of interhemispheric connectivity 2/2 stroke, normal pressure hydrocephalus

Vascular supply: ACA, MCA, PCA

6. Basal Ganglia (Fig. 2.5)

Anatomic borders: Collection of cell body nuclei enclosed by subcortical white matter and medially located

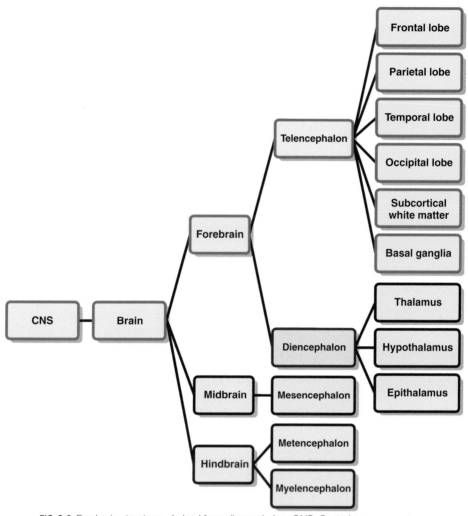

FIG. 2.6 Forebrain structures derived from diencephalon. *CNS*, Central nervous system.

Significance: Contains caudate, putamen, globus pallidus, subthalamic nucleus

Notable disease manifestations: Parkinson disease, Huntington disease, choreoathetosis 2/2 Wilson disease, Sydenham chorea 2/2 group A streptococcus, asterixis 2/2 hepatic encephalopathy, essential tremor, motor tics 2/2 Tourette

Vascular supply: Lenticulostriate branches of MCA

7. Thalamus (Figs. 2.6 and 2.7)

Anatomic location: Lateral wall of third ventricle

Significance: Contains myriad nuclei, including nuclei that process sensory input (VPL, VML, lateral geniculate,

QUICK TIPS

Diseases categorized as "Movement Disorders" are largely 2/2 basal ganglia pathology

QUICK TIPS

Striatum = caudate + putamen
Lenticular nucleus = putamen + globus pallidus

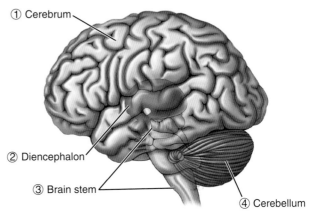

① Cerebrum

② Diencephalon

③ Brain stem

④ Cerebellum

FIG. 2.7 Diencephalon structures. (From Herlihy B, ed. *The Human Body in Health and Illness*. 4th ed. Philadelphia: Saunders; 2011.)

medial geniculate), motor output (VA, VL), and limbic connectivity (anterior, dorsomedial)

Notable disease manifestations: Dejerine-Roussy syndrome (aka thalamic pain syndrome)

Vascular supply: Branches of PCA

8. Hypothalamus

Anatomic location: Inferior to thalamus, anterior to brainstem

Significance: Contains suprachiasmatic nucleus (controls circadian rhythm), supraoptic nucleus (produces vasopressin), paraventricular nuclei (produces oxytocin), and arcuate nucleus (part of tuberoinfundibular pathway, secretes dopamine to regulate prolactin)

Notable disease manifestations: Wernicke-Korsakoff syndrome (mammillary body pathology), delayed sleep phase disorder, advanced sleep phase disorder, jet lag, shift work disorder, hyperprolactinemia 2/2 suppression of dopamine secretion, hypernatremia 2/2 decreased antidiuretic hormone (ADH) production

Vascular supply: Branches ACA, PCA, and basilar arteries

9. Epithalamus

Anatomic location: Posterior to thalamus

Significance: Contains pineal gland (releases melatonin)

Notable disease manifestations: Pinealoma

Vascular supply: branches of PCA

10. Limbic System (Fig. 2.8)

Anatomical location: A collection of medially located structures from both telencephalon and diencephalon

Significance: Homeostasis, Olfaction, Memory, Emotion; contains limbic cortex, hippocampus, amygdala,

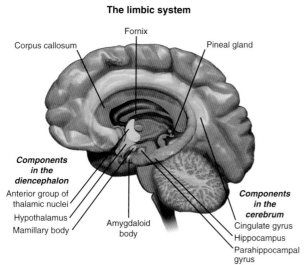

FIG. 2.8 Structures of the Limbic System. (Blausen.com staff. "Blausen gallery 2014." Wikiversity Journal of Medicine. https://en. wikiversity.org/wiki/Blausen_gallery_2014. http://dx.doi.org/10.15347/ wjm/2014.010. ISSN 20018762.)

olfactory cortex, hypothalamus, thalamus, habenula, basal ganglia, septal nuclei, basal forebrain, fornix, mammillary bodies

Notable disease manifestations: Kluver-Bucy syndrome, anterograde/retrograde amnesia, Wernicke-Korsakoff syndrome (2/2 mammillary body lesion)

Vascular supply: Branches of ACA, MCA, PCA

B. Midbrain (aka mesencephalon)

The midbrain consists of only one anatomic region and is derived only from the mesencephalon (making the two words interchangeable). Because the midbrain is the most superior aspect of the brainstem, it represents a transition from cortical and subcortical structures. To prepare for the shelf, learn the anatomy, function, and vascular supply of the midbrain.

1. Midbrain (aka mesencephalon) (Figs. 2.9 and 2.10)

Anatomic borders: Inferior to cerebral peduncles, superior to pons, anterior to cerebral aqueduct of Sylvius

Significance: Contains superior colliculus (visual), inferior colliculus (auditory), midbrain tectum (superior colliculus + inferior colliculus), cerebral peduncle, nuclei for CN3, nuclei for CN4, substantia nigra

Notable disease manifestations: Parinaud syndrome, Weber syndrome, Claude syndrome, and Parkinson disease (substantia nigra).

Vascular supply: PCA, basilar, paramedian arteries

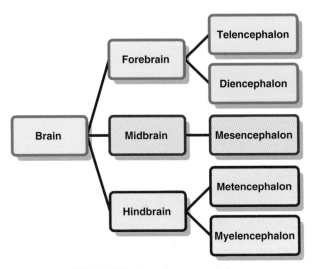

FIG. 2.9 Midbrain and mesencephalon.

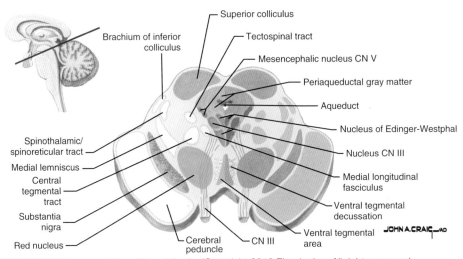

FIG. 2.10 Axial cross section of the midbrain. (Copyright 2016 Elsevier Inc. All rights reserved. http://www.netterimages.com.)

C. Hindbrain

The hindbrain consists of the metencephalon and the myelencephalon.

The metencephalon includes the pons and the cerebellum.

The myelencephalon includes just the medulla.

Shelf-worthy things to know about hindbrain principles include vascular supply, location of cranial nerve nuclei, and associated structures per level.

Hindbrain Structures Derived From the Metencephalon

1. Pons

Anatomic borders: Inferior to midbrain, superior to medulla, anterior to cerebellum

Significance: Contains nuclei for CN V, CN VI, CN VII, and CN VIII (CN 5–8)

Notable disease manifestations: Locked in syndrome, anterior inferior cerebellar artery (AICA) syndrome, lateral pontine syndrome

Vascular supply: AICA, superior cerebellar artery (SCA), paramedian branches of basilar artery

2. Cerebellum

Anatomic borders: Inferior to occipital lobe, posterior to pons

Significance: Contains lateral hemisphere (extremity motor planning), intermediate hemisphere (distal limb coordination), vermis, flocculonodular lobe, superior cerebellar peduncle (output), middle cerebral peduncle (input), inferior cerebellar peduncle (input)

Notable disease manifestations: Ataxia (ipsilateral to cerebellar region), truncal ataxia (2/2 vermis/flocculonodular aka midline pathology), appendicular ataxia (2/2 lateral pathology)

Vascular supply: SCA, AICA, posterior inferior cerebellar artery (PICA)

Hindbrain Structures Derived From the Myelencephalon

1. Medulla

Anatomic borders: Inferior to the pons, superior to C1 of the spinal cord

Significance: Contains nuclei for CN IX, CN X, CN XI, CN XII (CN 9–12)

Notable disease manifestations: Wallenberg syndrome (aka lateral medullary syndrome), medial medullary syndrome

Vascular supply: PICA, anterior spinal artery (ASA), paramedian branches of vertebral artery

Spinal Cord (Fig. 2.11)

The spinal cord is the other component of the CNS (in addition to the brain). It extends from the base of the medulla all the way down to the conus medullaris (which ends at the level of L2–L3). Spinal nerves below the conus medullaris are known as the cauda equina (horse's tail) and usually terminated from L3–L5. The spinal cord itself is covered by meninges (from external to internal: dura → arachnoid → pia), similar to the brain. Thus meningeal cover is one similarity that structures from the CNS share.

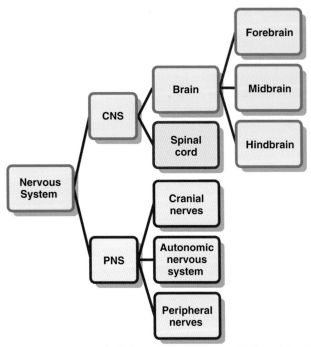

FIG. 2.11 Spinal cord. *CNS*, Central nervous system; *PNS*, peripheral nervous system.

For general principles, the key is to know the difference from conus medullaris and cauda equina (which can both lead to similar but distinct syndromes), as well as the organization of the vertebral column.

Of note, the spinal cord refers specifically to the tract of nerves that extends from C1 to L2–L3. The vertebral column refers to the bony vertebrae that protect the spinal cord and does not have any neuro connotations.

1. <u>Spinal Cord</u>

Anatomic location: C1 to L2–L3 of vertebral column (conus medullaris); runs through spinal canal and protected by vertebral column (aka spine).

Significance: Contains corticospinal, spinothalamic, and posterior column white matter tracts, cauda equina, conus medullaris, filum terminale.

Notable disease manifestations: Conus medullaris syndrome, cauda equina syndrome, Brown-Sequard syndrome, central cord syndrome 2/2 syringomyelia, spinal cord tumor; anterior cord syndrome 2/2 ASA infarct, trauma, myelitis

Vascular supply: ASAs, posterior spinal arteries

99 AR

Spinal arteries branch off different major vessels at different segments of the vertebra. Exact detail not necessary for shelf but if curious, please watch this tutorial

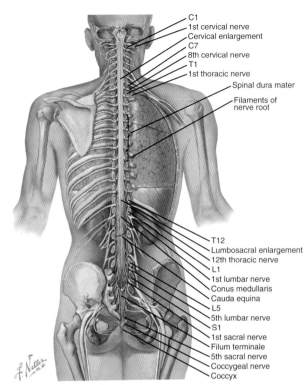

C1
1st cervical nerve
Cervical enlargement
C7
8th cervical nerve
T1
1st thoracic nerve
Spinal dura mater
Filaments of
nerve root

T12
Lumbosacral enlargement
12th thoracic nerve
L1
1st lumbar nerve
Conus medullaris
Cauda equina
L5
5th lumbar nerve
S1
1st sacral nerve
Filum terminale
5th sacral nerve
Coccygeal nerve
Coccyx

FIG. 2.12 Vertebral column and spinal cord. (Copyright 2016 Elsevier Inc. All rights reserved. http://www.netterimages.com.)

2. Vertebral Column (aka spine) (Fig. 2.12)

Anatomic location: A set of bones separated by cartilaginous joints that extends from cervical vertebra at the foramen magnum to the coccygeal vertebra in the pelvic area

Significance: Divided into five regions: cervical vertebral bodies (C1–C7), thoracic vertebrae (T1–T12), lumbar vertebrae (L1–L5), sacral vertebrae (S1–S5), coccygeal vertebra (Co1), nucleus pulposus, intervertebral discs

Notable disease manifestations: Slipped disc (e.g., lumbar disc herniation), spinal cord stenosis, spondylolisthesis, ankylosing spondylitis, rheumatoid arthritis of the cervical spine

Vascular supply: ASAs, posterior spinal arteries, segmental artery

Peripheral Nervous System

The PNS is the other half of the nervous system and can be conceptualized as the nerves that are projected from the previously covered CNS.

With regard to the shelf, understanding the normal function of cranial nerves, ANS, and spinal nerves that project from the spinal cord is important to answer questions about pathology. Although normal function itself won't be tested, knowledge of normal function is needed to decipher stem clues and exam findings within the question. Like the rest of the General Principles chapter, keep referring back to these sections if questions about normal arise in other readings of disease pathology.

Cranial Nerves (Fig. 2.13)

There are 12 cranial nerves, which can be categorized by both location and function with respect to the brainstem.

A helpful mnemonic is Gates' Rule of 4s: CN I–IV are located at or above the level of the midbrain; CN V–VIII are located at the level of the pons; and CN IX–XII are located at the level of the medulla [4].

With respect to function, cranial nerves can be motor, sensory, autonomic, or some mix of the three.

One helpful fact to remember are the four purely motor cranial nerves: CN III, IV, VI, XII (Tables 2.1–2.3). All four motor-only cranial nerves are located medially in their

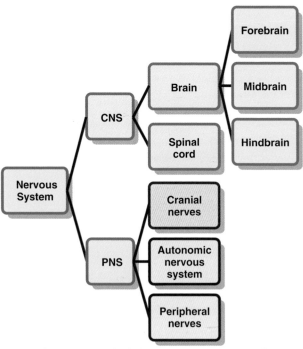

FIG. 2.13 Cranial nerves. *CNS*, Central nervous system; *PNS*, peripheral nervous system.

respective areas of the brainstem; only the IV nerve arises from the dorsal aspect of midbrain (Fig. 2.14). They can also all be remembered by being factors of 12 (since 3, 4, 6, and 12 are all divisible by 12).

Autonomic Nervous System

The ANS is composed of the (1) sympathetic division and (2) parasympathetic division.

For the shelf, know the normal functions of sympathetic and parasympathetic. Although you will not be asked about normal "fight-or-flight" and "rest-and-digest" processes, the clues given in a question stem may describe a normal autonomic process gone awry. Anticholinergic syndrome, for instance, presents as a patient in sympathetic overdrive.

TABLE 2.1 Cranial Nerves at or Above Level of Midbrain

	Location	Function	Key pathology
CN I, Olfactory Nerve	Olfactory bulb; olfactory nerves traverse cribriform plate of ethmoid bone	Sensory: Olfaction Motor: None Autonomic: None	Anosmia, Foster Kennedy syndrome
CN II, Optic Nerve	Optic nerve → optic tract → lateral geniculate nucleus of the thalamus	Sensory: Vision Motor: None Autonomic: None	Blindness
CN III, Oculomotor Nerve	Midbrain → levator palpebrae, medial rectus, inferior rectus, superior rectus, inferior oblique	Sensory: None Motor: Eyelid elevation, eye adduction, depression, elevation, extorsion Autonomic: parasympathetic pupil constrictor	"Blown pupil, down and out gaze" 2/2 uncal herniation
CN IV, Trochlear Nerve	Midbrain → superior oblique	Sensory: None Motor: depression and intorsion Autonomic: None	Inability to look down when descending stairs

TABLE 2.2 Cranial Nerves at or Above Level of the Pons

Cranial Nerve at the level of the pons	Location	Function	Key pathology
CN V, Trigeminal Nerve	Pons → masticator muscles, tensor tympani, tongue, face	Sensory: V1, V2, V3 divisions for pain, touch, temperature, position and vibration of face, mouth, anterior 2/3 tongue, meninges, nasal sinuses Motor: Muscles of mastication, tensor tympani Autonomic: None	Trigeminal neuralgia (tic douloureux), sensory loss ipsilateral to lesion
CN VI, Abducens Nerve	Pons → lateral rectus	Sensory: None Motor: Abduction of the eye Autonomic: None	Diplopia, inability to abduct eye
CN VII, Facial Nerve	Pons → muscles of facial expression, salivary glands, lacrimal glands, anterior 2/3 tongue, external auditory meatus	Sensory: pain, temp for external auditory meatus; taste for anterior 2/3 tongue Motor: facial expression muscles, stapedius, digastric Autonomic: parasympathetic → salivation, lacrimation	Bell palsy
CN VIII, Cochlear Nerve	Pons → cochlea	Sensory: Hearing, vestibular sensation Motor: None Autonomic: None	Sensorineural hearing loss, central vertigo, Meniere disease

Unlike Step 1, shelf questions do not require you to memorize the details of normal function. However, having a general sense of which processes are sympathetic and parasympathetic will help to diagnose disease.

Sympathetic Nervous System
Location: T1–L3 preganglionic neurons (acetylcholine) → sympathetic trunk, celiac ganglion, superior mesenteric

TABLE 2.3 Cranial Nerves at or Above the Level of the Medulla

Cranial Nerve at level of the medulla	Location	Function	Key pathology
CN IX, Glossopharyngeal Nerve	Medulla → stylopharyngeus muscle, parotid gland, middle ear, external auditory meatus, pharynx, posterior 1/3 tongue, carotid body	Sensory: **chemoreceptor** and **baroreceptor** of **carotid body**; taste and sensation for posterior 1/3 tongue, sensation for middle ear, external auditory meatus, pharynx. Motor: Stylopharyngeus muscle. Autonomic: **parasympathetic →** parotid gland	Loss of sensation, loss of BP regulation
CN X, Vagus Nerve	Medulla → pharyngeal/laryngeal muscles, heart, lungs, digestive tract, epiglottis, aortic arch	Sensory: **chemoreceptor/baroreceptor** of **aortic arch**; taste from epiglottis/pharynx, pharynx, external auditory meatus. Motor: Swallowing (pharyngeal muscles), Speech (laryngeal muscles). Autonomic: Parasympathetics from heart, lungs, and GI tract to splenic flexure	Hoarseness, dysphagia, lateral medullary syndrome
CN XI, Spinal Accessory Nerve	Medulla → sternocleidomastoid, trapezius	Sensory: None. Motor: Neck rotation (SCM), shrug (trapezius). Autonomic: None	Lateral medullary syndrome
CN XII, Hypoglossal Nerve	Midbrain → tongue	Sensory: None. Motor: tongue protrusion. Autonomic: None	Tongue deviation

ganglion, inferior mesenteric ganglion → target end organs (norepinephrine)

Function (from superior to inferior):

1. Dilates pupil
2. Inhibits salivation/lacrimation

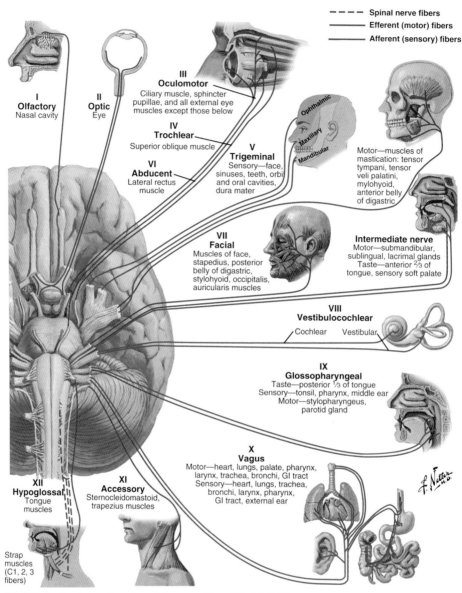

3. Dilates airways
4. Increases heart rate
5. Stimulates sweat gland secretion (only sympathetic process mediated through acetylcholine)
6. Piloerection
7. Digestion inhibition
8. Stimulates gluconeogenesis

9. Inhibits bile release
10. Constricts blood vessels in intestines (to redirect blood)
11. Relaxes urinary bladder
12. Ejaculation

Notable disease manifestations: Horner syndrome

Parasympathetic Nervous System (Fig. 2.15)

Location: CN III, VII, IX, X + S2-4 → parasympathetic ganglia in/near end organs → target end organs (completely acetylcholine mediated)

Function (from superior to inferior):

1. Constricts pupil
2. Stimulates salivation/lacrimation
3. Constricts airways
4. Decreases heart rate
5. Does not affect sweat secretion
6. Does not affect piloerection
7. Stimulates digestion
8. No effect on gluconeogenesis
9. Releases bile
10. Dilates blood vessels in intestines
11. Stimulates bladder contraction
12. Erection

Notable disease manifestations: Anticholinergic syndrome

Peripheral Nerves, Major Plexuses

For the purpose of the shelf exam, not all peripheral nerves are created equal. Questions on this topic predominantly cover branches of the brachial plexus and the lumbosacral plexus.

Be sure to know the general sensory and motor functions of the terminal nerves of these two major plexuses. For instance, with respect to the brachial plexus, memorizing the number of roots, trunks, divisions, and cords won't score you any extra points. However, knowing the sensory and motor function of the terminal branches of the brachial plexus (i.e., radial, median, ulnar, axillary, musculocutaneous nerves) will allow you to identify pathology on the question stem.

In particular, key in on unique features of each terminal nerve. For instance, if a patient in the question loses sensation only in the dorsal interweb space between the first and second toe, you can immediately identify an ipsilateral deep peroneal nerve lesion as the culprit (and without reading the rest of the question stem!).

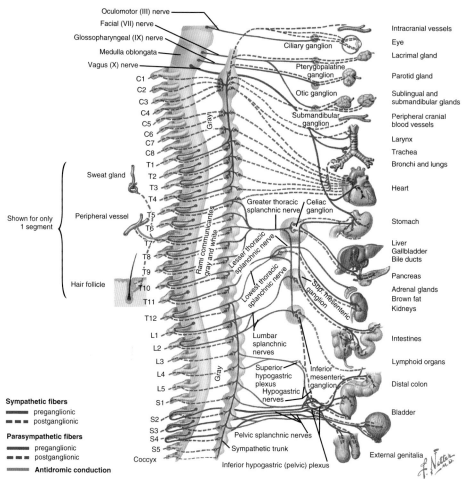

FIG. 2.15 Parasympathetic versus sympathetic nerves. (Copyright 2016 Elsevier Inc. All rights reserved. http://www.netterimages.com.)

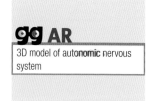

gg AR

3D model of autonomic nervous system

A. Brachial Plexus

1. Radial Nerve

Motor function: Extension of the arm, wrist, and proximal interphalangeal (PIP); forearm supination, thumb abduction

Sensory function: Posterior arm, forearm, dorsal lateral hand

Notable disease manifestations: Wrist drop, cheiralgia paresthetlca

2. Median Nerve

Motor function: Wrist flexion and abduction, forearm pronation, thumb, index, middle finger flexion; thumb opposition

Sensory: Thumb, index, middle, half of ring finger (ventral and dorsal sensation)

Notable disease manifestations: Carpal tunnel, preacher's hand, simian hand

3. <u>Ulnar Nerve</u>
Motor: Finger adduction and abduction, wrist flexion and
    adduction, flexion of ring finger and pinky
Sensory: ventral and dorsal pinky and half of ring finger
Notable disease manifestations: Ulnar claw
4. <u>Musculocutaneous Nerve</u>
Motor: Flexion of arm at elbow, supination of forearm
Sensory: Lateral Forearm
Notable disease manifestations: Numbness of lateral
    forearm
5. <u>Axillary Nerve</u>
Motor: Shoulder abduction beyond 15 degrees
Sensory: Deltoid
Notable disease manifestations: Numbness of deltoid/
    shoulder

B. **Lumbosacral Plexus**
1. <u>Femoral Nerve</u>
Motor: Flexion at hip, extension at knee
Sensory: Anterior thigh, medial leg
Notable disease manifestations: Ulnar claw
2. <u>Obturator Nerve</u>
Motor: Thigh adduction
Sensory: Medial thigh
Notable disease manifestations: Numbness of medial thigh
3. <u>Sciatic Nerve</u>
Motor: Flexion at knee
Sensory: Posterior leg and ventral/dorsal foot
Notable disease manifestations: The sciatic nerve itself
    branches into tibial and peroneal nerves; thus, the sci-
    atic nerve branches rather than the sciatic nerve itself
    will be tested on the shelf
4. <u>Tibial Nerve</u> (branch of sciatic)
Motor: Foot plantar flexion, inversion, toe flexion
Sensory: Dorsum and lateral aspect of foot
Notable disease manifestations: Inability to plantar flex
    and invert foot
5. <u>Superficial peroneal</u> (branch of common peroneal from
    sciatic)
Motor: Foot eversion
Sensory: Lateral leg and foot, dorsum of foot except for
    first/second toe interweb space
Notable disease manifestations: Loss of eversion
6. <u>Deep Peroneal Nerve</u> (branch of common peroneal
    from sciatic)
Motor: Foot dorsiflexion, toe extension
Sensory: First/second interweb toe space on dorsum of foot

Notable disease manifestations: Loss of sensation on first/second interweb toes space on dorsum of foot

Miscellaneous General Principle Topics

This section focuses on the types of questions that one can expect to see of the "General Principle" variety on the shelf. Remember, this accounts for only 1%–5% of the exam. Most likely, it will be a question about normal aging.

Vascular supply of the brain and neuroimaging principles are also useful to know.

A. Normal Aging

Buzz Words: Decreased Achilles tendon reflex (aka "1+" or less) + difficulty remembering if not enough rest + awakens early in the morning + increasing stiffness + presbyopia + presbycusis → normal aging

Clinical Presentation: As mentioned in the intro, know how to spot a patient who is aging appropriately for her or his age. The classic example is a >65-year-old patient coming in for a regular health maintenance exam with 1+ Achilles reflex and sleeping less with no real chief complaint. [Gunner Goggles 1+ Achilles reflex + older individual + everything else is within realm of normal → normal aging]

PPx: N/A

MoD: N/A

Dx: N/A

Tx/Mgmt: N/A

GUNNER PRACTICE

1. An 80-year-old woman comes in for a health maintenance examination. She states that she occasionally has difficulty remembering the names of her friends when she does not sleep well. She also reports waking early in the morning and increasing stiffness with walking over the past 10 years. She takes hydrochlorothiazide for hypertension and presented with a blood pressure of 138/88 mm Hg. Physical and mental status examinations reveal no abnormalities. Which is the most likely cause of this patient's symptoms?

A. Dementia, Alzheimer type

B. Normal Aging

C. Medication adverse effect

D. Parkinson disease

E. Multiinfarct (vascular) dementia

Notes

ANSWERS: What Would Gunner Jess/Jim Do?

1. WWGJD? An 80-year-old woman comes in for a health maintenance examination. She states that she occasionally has difficulty remembering the names of her friends when she does not sleep well. She also reports waking early in the morning and increasing stiffness with walking over the past 10 years. She takes hydrochlorothiazide for hypertension and presented with a blood pressure of 138/88 mm Hg. Physical and mental status examinations reveal no abnormalities. Which is the most likely cause of this patient's symptoms?

Answer: B, Normal Aging

Explanation: Patient has no clear chief complaint. The question stem states that physical and mental status examinations are normal, which increase suspicion for normal aging. In addition, decreased memory in old age is normal. It becomes pathologic only when decrease in memory impairs function.

A. Dementia, Alzheimer type → Incorrect. Don't be fooled by the statement "she occasionally has difficulty remembering the names of her friends." Her memory lapses are only occasional, and there is no other indication that this impairs her daily function. The biggest giveaway is that the mental status exam was normal. If the patient had Alzheimer disease, the mini mental status exam (MMSE) would by definition be at least below a 27/30 (or abnormal).

C. Medication adverse effect → Incorrect. The only medication that is listed or inferred is hydrochlorothiazide (HCTZ). In general, "medication adverse effect" is only the answer if onset of symptoms coincides with taking the medication. However, because the timeline of when patient started taking HCTZ is ambiguous and memory deficits are not a typical side effect, this answer can also be ruled out.

D. Parkinson disease → Incorrect. Parkinson disease will typically present with resting tremor, cogwheel rigidity, shuffling of feet (or at the very least an abnormal physical exam). This patient's normal physical exam findings rules this answer out.

E. Multiinfarct (vascular) dementia → Incorrect. The classic question stem for a patient suffering multiinfarct dementia is one whose memory deteriorates subacutely (over the course of several months) but becomes progressively worse. This patient's inability to remember names of friends is not progressive and does not have a subacute timeline; therefore, ruling this answer choice out.

Psychiatry in the Clinical Neurology Shelf

Hao-Hua Wu, Leo Wang, and Chuang-Kuo Wu

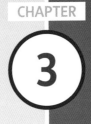

Aside from internal medicine, psychiatry and neurology have the largest overlap for shelf content. This chapter will highlight only the psychiatry topics that most frequently appear, including disorders leading to visual/olfactory hallucinations, adjustment disorder, major depressive disorder (MDD), conversion disorder, and alcohol intoxication/ withdrawal.

Because this is only 3%–7% of the test, skip the Mental Disorders chapter if you are pressed for time or have already done your psych rotation. If you still need a psych refresher, spend no more than 1 hour before moving on to the next chapter.

Hallucination and Related Disorders

For the purposes of the neuro shelf, be familiar with the definitions of and the differences between **(1) hallucination, (2) illusion, (3) psychosis,** and **(4) delusion.** These are all mental status exam findings that include neurologic disease in the differential. Know how to differentiate neurologic and psychiatric disease.

A. Hallucination: **Patient experiences sensory perception with** no stimulus **(vs. illusion, in which patient misinterprets a** real stimulus**)**
   - Hallucinations are organized by the five senses

1. **Delirium** (visual hallucination) (Table 3.1)

Buzz Words: Waxing and waning + sundowning + recent surgery or change in treatment regimen + abnormal electroencephalogram (EEG) + >65-year-old patient + anticholinergic med + not alert on mental exam

Clinical Presentation: Patients with delirium have fluctuating mental status (vs. dementia, which is nonfluctuating). It is typically acute onset versus schizophrenia, which is 6 months. A key feature is sundowning, in which the symptoms get worse at night. Patients also will exhibit impaired consciousness and attention, visual/tactile hallucinations, and agitation.

PPx: (1) Let the patient sleep comfortably through the night (no 5 a.m. labs), (2) stop unnecessary meds, decrease

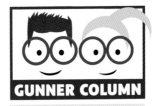

QUICK TIPS

Neuroanatomic Psych Correlates

Enlargement of cerebral ventricles → schizophrenia, NPH

Decreased hippocampal volume → posttraumatic stress disorder, Alzheimer

Decreased volume of amygdala → panic disorder!

OCD → Orbitofrontal cortex and striatum

Increased total brain volume → autism

QUICK TIPS

Illusion example: interpreting somebody's whisper as a scream or interpreting someone's touch as a slap. Unlikely that illusion symptoms will show up on shelf but useful for better understanding hallucination.

QUICK TIPS

The KEY to recognizing delirium vs. dementia is that delirium is **acute** and **waxes and wanes**.

TABLE 3.1 Types of Hallucination

Hallucination type (in order of relevance to neuro shelf)	Definition	Neuro disease manifestation
Olfactory Hallucination	Smelling something that isn't there	Seizure
Visual Hallucination	Seeing something that isn't there	Delirium, Lewy body dementia, PCP and LSD intoxication; alcohol/benzo withdrawal
Tactile Hallucination	Feeling something that isn't there	Alcohol withdrawal, cocaine or amphetamine intoxication
Auditory hallucination	Hearing something that isn't there	N/A → **Always psych related**
Gustatory hallucination	Tasting something that isn't there	N/A

stimuli, and (3) orient the patient to room with calendar and clock

MoD: Exact mechanism unknown but can be precipitated by any insult, including meds (benzos, anticholinergics), alcohol withdrawal, meningitis, poison, etc.

Dx:

1. Mental status examination
2. Head magnetic resonance imaging (MRI) or computed tomography (CT) to rule out stroke or subdural hematoma
3. EEG to rule out epileptic activity
4. UA, blood culture, glucose, BMP, B12, RPR (to look for cause)

Tx/Mgmt:

1. PPx against delirium (let patient sleep, stop meds, decrease stimuli, orient patient to room with calendar/clock
2. Haloperidol, quetiapine to calm agitation in elderly
3. Benzos in young patients OK
   - Avoid benzos in elderly because they could exacerbate symptoms (Sx)

2. **Lewy Body Dementia** (LBD)

Buzz Words: Benign visual hallucinations ("Lilliputian" pleasant hallucinations) + visuospatial dysfunction + **memory loss** + Sx of Parkinsonism (bradykinesia, tremor, rigidity, abnormal posture)

Clinical Presentation: LBD is high-yield because of its distinct Buzz Words in the setting of memory loss (e.g., Lilliputian hallucinations). If dementia >12 months, Parkinson disease with dementia (see later). Patients present with parkinsonian symptoms (bradykinesia, tremor, abnormal posture, rigidity) and dementia (dementia may precede or follow parkinsonian symptoms). Visual hallucinations and rapid eye movement (REM) sleep behavior disorders are often seen.

PPx: None

MoD: Degeneration of dopamine releasing neurons in basal ganglia, substantia nigra pars compacta; intracytoplasmic alpha-synuclein inclusions in neocortex and midbrain dopaminergic cells

Dx:
1. MMSE
2. MRI to rule out vascular dementia
3. UDS to rule out medication toxicity

Tx/Mgmt:
1. Treat parkinsonian features with levo-carbidopa (but may lead to worsening hallucinations/delirium).
2. Treat cognitive symptoms with acetylcholinesterase inhibitors (donepezil)
   - Dopaminergic agonists often trigger visual hallucinations and psychotic behaviors
   - Hypersensitivity to antipsychotics

B. Psychosis: **Break from reality with delusions, perceptual disturbances, or disordered thought; EEG is normal**
   - Behavioral presentation of delusions and hallucinations linked with thought disorders

   Examples of psychotic disorders: Schizophrenia, brief psychotic disorder, schizophreniform, schizoaffective disorder
   - These disorders won't be directly tested but may show up as an answer choice
   - Do not confuse with delirium, because delirious patients have an abnormal EEG and are not psychotic

C. Delusions: **Fixed false belief that persists; bizarre versus nonbizarre**
   Example of delusional disorders: Delusional disorder, schizophrenia
   - Like psychotic disorders, won't be directly tested but may show up as an answer choice.

Anxiety and Related Disorders

It is unlikely that anxiety disorders will be tested directly. However, you may see several anxiety-related disorders pop up as answer choices (such as adjustment disorder), so it's good to separate anxiety-related from mood-related problems.

A. Adjustment Disorder (Begins <3 months after the stressor and ends <6 months after stressor)

Buzz Words: <3 months onset from **identifiable** stressor + stress not life-threatening (vs. posttraumatic stress disorder [PTSD]) + stressor not 2/2 lost loved one (vs. bereavement) + anxious and/or "depressed" but patient states that he/she can still enjoy hobbies

- If patient has anhedonia (inability to experience joy), rule out adjustment disorder → more likely MDD
- If symptoms last >6 months → general anxiety disorder
- If symptoms last >6 months and stressor recurs → chronic adjustment disorder
- If loss of a loved one + Sx <2 months → bereavement; >1 year of bereavement = pathologic grief

Clinical Presentation: Adjustment disorder is characterized by emotional or behavioral symptoms (e.g., anxiety, depression, disturbance of conduct) that develop **within 3 months** in response to an **identifiable stressor** and **last no longer than 6 months after the stressor ends.** It is on the spectrum of anxiety disorders. Adjustment disorder can be differentiated from acute stress disorder and PTSD by **its lack of a life-threatening trauma.**

PPx: None

MoD: Increased norepinephrine, decreased serotonin, decreased GABA

Dx: Mental status exam

Tx/Mgmt (not necessary for neuro shelf):

1. Psychotherapy
2. Benzos for insomnia or to control anxiety
   - Take home point is that you do NOT treat adjustment disorder with selective serotonin reuptake inhibitors (SSRIs)

Mood Disorders

Depression is the most commonly tested psych disorder in the neurology shelf. Know how to recognize it and differentiate it from adjustment disorder, dysthymia, and bipolar disorder.

A. Major Depressive Disorder (≥2 weeks)

Buzz Words: Sadness, anhedonia ≥2 weeks (5/9 SIGECAPS sx) + no evidence of medication use + no evidence dementia → MDD

- If >2 years → dysthymia
- If depression with episodes of mania → bipolar I

Clinical Presentation: MDD can occur at any age with a chief complaint of one of the SIGECAPS symptoms, such as difficulty concentrating, in the setting of dysfunction at work or home. The most specific symptom of MDD on the shelf is anhedonia. Be on the lookout for the timing of symptoms (has to meet five out of nine SIGECAPS symptoms for at least 2 weeks), as well as any concomitant symptoms. If patient also has psychotic symptoms, MDD with psychotic features and schizoaffective disorder is also on the differential.

PPx: None

MoD: Neurotransmitter deficiencies in brain and CSF of serotonin, Decreased 5-HIAA and serotonin in CSF; may also have decreased dopamine and NE

Dx:

1. Mental status exam
2. UDS to rule out substance use (e.g., stimulant withdrawal, opiates) and medication use (e.g., propranolol)
3. Head CT/MRI to rule out stroke, other medical causes
4. Positron emission tomography may show decreased blood flow in b/l frontal lobes

Tx/Mgmt (not necessary for neuro shelf):

1. Assess for suicidal ideation
2. SSRIs and TCAs → 70%
3. MAOIs if refractory or atypical
4. ECT if 2–3 failed medical trials, severe suicidality, catatonia, malnutrition

Somatoform and Factitious Disorders

Somatoform and factitious disorders, especially conversion disorder, occasionally show up on the shelf. It is important to know the definitions of the following:

Somatoform: Patients believe they are ill

Factitious: Patients pretend they are ill with internal incentives

Malingering: Patients pretend they are ill with external incentives

In addition, be familiar with conversion disorder, Munchausen, and malingering.

99 AR

SIGECAPS

A. Conversion Disorder (resolution in 1 month)

Buzz Words: At least one pseudoneuro finding (e.g., shifting paralysis or seizures or mutism) + psych trigger + not due to general medical cause + impairs function + unaware of symptoms, la belle indifference → conversion disorder

- If patient is aware of pseudoneuro symptoms → somatization (as patients suffering from conversion are typically unaware)

Clinical Presentation: Patients with conversion disorder act **indifferent** to the fact that they have some sort of neurologic dysfunction. This phenomenon is la belle indifference. No other disorder presents this way.

PPx: None

MoD: None

Dx:

1. Head CT/MRI to rule out brain pathology
2. BMP
3. CBC
4. UA
5. UDS

Tx/Mgmt (not necessary for neuro shelf):

1. Symptoms resolve after hypnosis or amobarbital
2. Insight oriented psychotherapy

B. Factitious Disorder (aka Munchausen)

Buzz Words: Patient intentionally harming self (i.e., insulin injection to appear hypoglycemic) + no external incentives → factitious disorder

- If child → Munchausen by proxy (adult is causing child's illness)

Clinical Presentation: The two types of factitious disorders are factitious disorder imposed on self and factitious disorder imposed on another. Both of these conditions involve faking a medical illness (either physical or mental) to assume the role of the patient. In factitious disorder imposed on self, the person assumes the patient role, whereas in factitious disorder imposed on another, the person fabricates a condition in someone under his or her care. This is most commonly seen in elderly patients or children.

Factitious disorders can be differentiated from malingering by the purpose of faking the illness. In malingering, there is a tangible gain (i.e., monetary compensation, time off work), whereas in factitious disorder the primary intent is psychological gain. This disorder is often seen in medical professionals, who know how to fake the condition accurately.

PPx: N/A
MoD: N/A
Dx: N/A
Tx/Mgmt:
1. Avoid unnecessary procedures
2. Screen for history of abuse in patient
3. Establish therapeutic alliance, treat with psychotherapy
4. Screen for comorbid borderline personality disorder

C. Malingering

Buzz Words: Patient intentionally harming self (i.e., insulin injection to appear hypoglycemic) + clear external incentive (e.g., criminal avoiding jail) → malingering

Clinical Presentation: Patients who malinger on the shelf are often nonmedical personnel who have a clear secondary gain. Patients with factitious disorder are usually medical personnel who fake symptoms with no obvious secondary gain.

PPx: N/A
MoD: N/A
Dx: N/A
Tx/Mgmt:
1. Treat medical problems as needed
2. Avoid unnecessary procedures
3. Establish therapeutic alliance, treat with psychotherapy

Substance Abuse Disorders

Due to its prevalence and broad clinical presentation, substance abuse disorders are a commonly tested shelf topic. For the neuro shelf, know the presentation of alcohol intoxication and withdrawal.

A. Alcohol Intoxication

Buzz Words: Disinhibition + ataxia + sedation + respiratory depression → acute alcoholic intoxication
Altered mental status, ophthalmoplegia, ataxia (AOA) → Wernicke syndrome
AOA + confabulation, amnesia, and psychomotor agitation (CAPA) → Korsakoff

Clinical Presentation: See Buzz Words
PPx: Counseling
MoD: EtOH is a GABA agonist and glutamate antagonist
• Mammillary body atrophy → Wernicke-Korsakoff syndrome

Dx:
1. Breathalyzer
2. Blood alcohol content (BAC)

3. Elevated GGT
4. 2/4 CAGE questionnaire with eye-opener most sensitive
5. Carbohydrate-deficient transferrin (CDT)
6. Head CT/MRI

Tx/Mgmt:
1. Only supportive treatment (or gastric lavage) unless there is dependence.
2. If there is dependence, treat as you would a withdrawal

B. Alcohol Withdrawal

Buzz Words: (Within 24 hours) Insomnia + Anxiety + Tachycardia + Nausea + Tremors + AVTH while alert and oriented + Seizures + delirium tremens (72 hours) + visual/tactile hallucinations

Clinical Presentation: See Buzz Words

PPx: Prevent by treating alcohol dependence. (1) Alcoholics Anonymous (2) naltrexone (mu receptor antagonist), disulfiram (acetaldehyde DH inhibitor), acamprosate, topiramate (reduces alcohol cravings), (3) rehab

MoD: Overinhibition of GABA

Dx:
1. Physical exam
2. CIWA score
3. Hyperreflexia to dose benzos during treatment if patient taking beta-blockers to mask withdrawal symptoms

Tx/Mgmt:
1. Thiamine first (with folate)
2. Diazepam and chlordiazepoxide if good liver function (long acting); glucuronidated + oxidated in liver
3. Lorazepam, temazepam, oxazepam if poor liver function, only glucuronidated in the liver
4. Mg^{2+} for seizures

GUNNER PRACTICE

1. A 27-year-old woman has felt depressed and stressed since returning to her job as a lawyer after the birth of her third child 4 years ago. She also has decreased energy and has lost interest in things she used to enjoy. However, there have not been any changes in fatigue, sleep, or weight. She does not take any medication and denies alcohol and drug use. Physical exam is within normal limits. On mental status exam, she is engaging with a full range of affect. There is no evidence of psychosis or suicidal ideation. What is the most likely diagnosis?
   A. Bipolar disorder 1
   B. Schizoaffective disorder

C. Adjustment disorder
D. Dysthymic disorder
E. Major depressive disorder

2. A 39-year-old woman presents to her physician with several complaints. She has a 25-year history of multiple symptoms, which have included headaches, pain in her back, arms, neck, legs, nausea, vomiting, diarrhea, constipation, sexual dysfunction, and urinary urgency. She has seen multiple physicians since she was 13. Which of the following is the most appropriate statement by the physician?
   A. "I'd like to run a series of tests to evaluate you for porphyria."
   B. "I think you may be malingering."
   C. "Your symptoms could be caused by stress. I would like for you to see a psychiatrist."
   D. "Tell me about any emotional trauma you may have experienced during childhood."
   E. "I would like to assess the symptoms that cause you the most distress and schedule a follow-up appointment."

3. An intoxicated 21-year-old college student is brought to the emergency room after sustaining a humoral fracture after a fall from the roof of her college sorority house. Two days after internal fixation, she is agitated, confused, and demands to leave the hospital against medical advice. She claims that she has an exam, although it is a Sunday. She accuses the nurses of torturing her. Her pulse is 126/min, and blood pressure is 150/100 mm Hg. She is diaphoretic. Which of the following best explains her behavior?
   A. Alcohol intoxication
   B. Alcohol withdrawal delirium
   C. Bipolar disorder
   D. Delusional disorder
   E. Posttraumatic stress disorder

ANSWERS: What Would Gunner Jess/Jim Do?

1. **WWGJD?** A 27-year-old woman has felt **depressed and stressed since** returning to her job as a lawyer after the birth of her third child **4 years ago.** She also has decreased energy and has **lost interest in things she used to enjoy.** However, there have **not been any changes in** fatigue, **sleep,** or weight. She does not take any medication and denies alcohol and drug use. Physical exam is within normal limits. On mental status exam, she is engaging with a full range of affect. There is **no evidence of psychosis** or suicidal ideation. What is the most likely diagnosis?

   Answer: D, Dysthymic disorder

   Explanation: Patient has the two key Buzz Words that point to depression: (1) sadness (aka "depressed and stressed") and (2) anhedonia ("lost interest in things she used to enjoy"). That should narrow down the possible answer choices to D (dysthymic disorder) and E (major depression). Both dysthymic disorder and major depression have similar presentations. The only difference is timeline. Major depression can be officially diagnosed 2 weeks after onset of symptoms and should resolve by 2 years. If symptoms of depression continue past 2 years, then the patient is diagnosed as officially having "dysthymic disorder." Because these symptoms have been ongoing for the past "4 years," or more than 2 years, the correct answer is dysthymic disorder. A key point to this question is recognizing that duration of symptoms is the key to solving questions pertaining to psych disorders. Other things to recognize is that she is on no medications or substance use. It is also important to note that there is "no evidence of psychosis" because that rules out other psychotic disorders like schizoaffective and schizophrenia.

   A. Bipolar disorder 1 → Incorrect. Bipolar disorder 1 is characterized by full episodes of mania in addition to lulls of depression. The patient here does not exhibit any of the Buzz Words of mania, such as sleepless nights, flight of ideas, and grandiosity of speech.

   B. Schizoaffective disorder → Incorrect. Schizoaffective disorder is characterized by mood abnormalities (e.g., mania or depression) in the context of underlying psychosis. Although the patient does have depressed mood, as evidenced by her abulia, she does not exhibit psychosis.

   C. Adjustment disorder → Incorrect. Again, this can be ruled out by timeline. Adjustment disorder by definition ends within 6 months from time of stressor. If it goes past 6 months, it is known as general anxiety disorder. Another important thing to remember is that adjustment disorder is on the spectrum of anxiety disorders and not mood disorders.

E. Major Depressive Disorder → Incorrect. By definition, MDD has to resolve 2 years from the onset of symptoms. If the symptoms have been going past 2 years, then it is identified as dysthymic disorder.

2. WWGJD? A 39-year-old woman presents to her physician with several complaints. She has a 25-year history of multiple symptoms, which have included headaches, pain in her back, arms, neck, legs, nausea, vomiting, diarrhea, constipation, sexual dysfunction, and urinary urgency. She has seen multiple physicians since she was 13. Which of the following is the most appropriate statement by the physician?

Answer: E, "I would like to assess the symptoms that cause you the most distress and schedule a follow-up appointment."

This is a classic presentation of a somatoform disorder, wherein patients, usually women, will present with a series of unexplained symptoms that are not consistent with physical exam or lab findings. This does not mean these patients do not experience these symptoms, though. On the shelf, the best management for somatoform disorders is to provide them access to physicians with consistent follow-up appointments. When a patient presents with symptoms despite abnormal findings, always think about somatoform, factitious disorders, or malingering. Typically, a plethora of symptoms that includes **sexual dysfunction** will suggest somatoform, whereas a single symptom or two will suggest fictitious or malingering.

A. "I'd like to run a series of tests to evaluate you for porphyria." → Incorrect. Never order more lab tests for someone with a somatoform disorder. This can only exacerbate her existing condition.

B. "I think you may be malingering." → There is no evidence she is malingering given that there are no external gains to be had by her particular illness. Moreover, malingering patients typically present more acutely and do not have the extensive medical history that somatoform disorders have.

C. "Your symptoms could be caused by stress. I would like for you to see a psychiatrist." → Although stress is certainly related to somatoform disorders, you should never trivialize the symptoms that a somatoform patient feels by claiming their symptoms are in their head.

D. "Tell me about any emotional trauma you may have experienced during childhood." → There is no evidence to suggest that there was a history of emotional trauma.

3. WWGJD? An intoxicated 21-year-old college student is brought to the emergency room after sustaining a humeral fracture after a fall from the roof of her college sorority house. Two days after open reduction internal fixation, she is agitated, confused, and demands to leave the hospital against medical advice. She claims that she has an exam, although it is a Sunday. She accuses the nurses of torturing her. Her pulse is 126/min, and blood pressure is 150/100 mm Hg. She is diaphoretic. Which of the following best explains her behavior?

Answer: B, Alcohol withdrawal

Explanation: Alcohol withdrawal is a frequently tested shelf topic that you should know like the back of your hand. Look for tremors, anxiety, tachycardia, and diaphoresis. This can often affect orientation and cause patients to be delirious with or without hallucinations. Her claims of having an exam and that the nurses are torturing her suggest she is confused and not oriented to time.

A. Alcohol intoxication → Acute alcohol intoxication is unlikely in this patient given that her symptoms are present 2 days after hospital admission.

C. Bipolar disorder 1 → Although she may be bipolar, the acute presentation without the history suggests otherwise. In addition, psychiatric disorders cannot be diagnosed in the setting of substance use.

D. Delusional disorder → Delusional disorder is usually persistent for longer than just a hospital stay. Usually these patients have an odd belief that is generally inconsistent with other areas of their life.

E. Posttraumatic stress disorder → Although she could eventually develop posttraumatic stress disorder, it takes 6 months for her to meet official diagnostic criteria.

Disorders of the Special Senses

Diana Kim, Hao-Hua Wu, Leo Wang, and Chuang-Kuo Wu

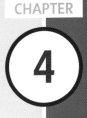

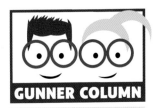

GUNNER COLUMN

Of the four special senses (visual, auditory, gustatory, and olfactory) only disorders of the eye and ear will be tested on the neurology shelf. While there will not be many direct questions about the eye and ear, many neurologic disorders present with eye and ear signs and symptoms. For instance, stroke may present with visual disturbances, and the National Board of Medical Examiners (NBME) may try to trick you with answer choices that reflect disorders of the retina or optic nerve.

General Disorders of the Eye

Luckily for test-takers, the eye is not a major focus of the neurology shelf despite a plethora of content; this is because most of these topics will fall into the scope of ophthalmology. However, a basic understanding of some of the most common and debilitating eye diseases is still necessary. The most important underlying principle in this chapter is timing of disease. Diseases that develop over long periods of time (age-related macular degeneration [ARMD]) are very different from those that occur acutely (retinal detachment). The most commonly tested acute eye disease is retinal detachment. The three most testable chronic diseases in this chapter are glaucoma, cataracts, and ARMD. A basic understanding of their pathophysiology, diagnosis (Dx), and basic treatment is enough to answer any question the NBME can throw at you.

A. Refractive Disorders (Presbyopia, Myopia, Hyperopia, Astigmatism)

Buzz Words:
- Young patient + difficulty seeing classroom whiteboard + age-appropriate complaints → myopia
- Older people + difficulty reading books without glasses + age appropriate complaints → hyperopia

Clinical Presentation: Refractive errors are the most frequent eye problems in the United States. Refractive errors include myopia (nearsightedness), hyperopia (farsightedness), astigmatism (distorted vision at all

> **QUICK TIPS**
> Refractive disorders are associated with normal (e.g., age-appropriate, nonpathologic) complaints.

distances), and presbyopia, which occur between age 40 and 50 years. On the shelf, this presents in activities of daily living. Patients may report an inability to read letters of the phone book and a need to hold a newspaper farther away to see clearly. Refractive disorders are corrected by eyeglasses, contact lenses, or in some cases, surgery. Although these topics are imperative to patient care, luckily most of these details fall into the scope of optometry and are thus not imperative to the exam. The most important takeaway from this section is identifying the common presentations for refractive disorders and *recognizing the difference* between them and other, more serious eye disorders. The latter is more commonly tested, but an understanding of the former is needed to triage answer choices.

PPx: None

MoD:

- Myopia (nearsightedness): eye is too long or lens is too curved → focuses light in front of retina
- Hyperopia (farsightedness): eye is too short or lens is too flat → focuses light behind retina
- Astigmatism: corneal curvature → imperfect refraction or focus that can occur with either hyperopia or myopia

Dx:

1. Ophthalmic/optometric evaluation
2. Automated refraction

Tx/Mgmt:

1. Eyeglasses/contacts
2. LASIK

QUICK TIPS

Cataract symptoms are exacerbated at night.

B. Cataracts

Buzz Words:

- Gradual onset + >40 years old (y/o) + faded colors, blurry vision, halos around light, trouble with bright lights, and trouble seeing at night + trouble driving, reading, or recognizing faces + otherwise normal history

Clinical Presentation: A cataract is a common disease in which the lens becomes opaque. It occurs after the age of 40. Presentation of cataracts earlier than the typical timeframe should raise suspicion for an underlying genetic disorder, such as Lowe syndrome and neurofibromatosis type 2. The trickiest part of cataracts is differentiating them from other diseases that may present similarly. Usually on the exam, the giveaway will be patients with problems occurring at **night** when the translucency of the lens is most imperative because there is less light. The patient also will not have other pathologic complaints. Most cataracts are easily diagnosed and completely curable, so they are a relatively easy disease to manage for ophthalmologists.

PPx: (1) Decrease preventable risk factors (UVB exposure and smoking); (2) diabetes management; (3) vitamins A, C, and E supplementation; (4) lutein and zeaxanthin supplementation; (5) statins

MoD:
- Oxidation and glycation damage of lens, crystalline crosslinking → opacification of lens = cataracts

Dx:
1. Blood glucose
2. Slit-lamp eye exam

Tx/Mgmt:
1. Treat medical causes
2. Cataract surgery
3. Phacoemulsification

C. Glaucoma (Open and Closed Angle)

Buzz Words:
- Frequent eyeglass lens changes + mild headaches + visual disturbances + impaired adaption to darkness (but can be asymptomatic until late) + gradual loss of peripheral vision + cupping of optic nerve on fundoscope → open-angle glaucoma
- Extreme eye pain + blurred vision + headache + nausea and vomiting + red eye + pupil is dilated and nonreactive to light + acute onset + onset of symptoms in a movie theater (dark room) → closed-angle glaucoma

Clinical Presentation: Glaucoma is a commonly tested disease defined by damage to the optic nerve and vision loss. In the eye, aqueous humor produced by the ciliary body of the iris travels through the pupil into the anterior chamber and is then drained via the trabecular meshwork in the angle of the anterior chamber. Any process that disrupts this natural flow can ↑ intraocular pressure (IOP), damage the optic nerve, and cause visual field deficits. Glaucoma is the result of such damage to the nerve. For the purposes of the shelf, glaucoma is divided into two main categories: "open-angle" and "closed-angle" glaucoma, which describe mechanisms by which IOP increases. A third category, "normal-tension glaucoma," exists but is not tested.

QUICK TIPS
MoD cataracts more likely Step 1 than a shelf question.

QUICK TIPS
Open-angle glaucoma presents gradually on the shelf. Closed-angle presents acutely.

QUICK TIPS
Closed-angle classically presents in a dark room 2/2 pupillary dilation.

Open-angle chronic glaucoma is painless, tends to develop slowly over time, and often has no symptoms until the disease has progressed significantly. Closed-angle glaucoma is chronic and asymptomatic in some cases, but can also present acutely out of nowhere. Closed-angle symptoms include sudden eye pain, blurred vision, a dilated pupil, redness, nausea, and vomiting, resulting from a sudden spike in IOP from iridotrabecular contact. Acute, closed-angle glaucoma is an ophthalmologic emergency. Glaucoma, both open and closed, can permanently damage vision in the affected eye, first by decreasing peripheral vision (reducing the visual field), and then potentially leading to blindness if left untreated. In terms of the treatment, the types of drugs used to treat open- and closed-angle glaucoma are fair game for the neurology shelf!

PPx: (1) Frequent eye checks, (2) exercise and eye protection among other preventable risk factors, (3) laser peripheral iridotomy, which creates a hole in the peripheral iris, as PPx for closed-angle glaucoma in those with open-angle glaucoma

MoD:
- Damage to retinal ganglion cells from increased IOP → visual field deficits and can occur via open or closed mechanisms
- Open angle: flow of aqueous humor is decreased through trabecular meshwork from diabetes or genetic causes (AAs) → elevated IOP
- Closed angle: Iris dilates → pushes against the lens of the eye → disrupted flow of aqueous humor into anterior chamber → pressure in the posterior chamber pushes the iris forward, blocks angle

Dx:
- Closed angle: (1) clinical history and (2) eye examination
- Open angle: (1) tonometry, (2) ophthalmoscopic visualization of the optic nerve, and (3) visual field testing

Tx/Mgmt:
- **Closed Angle:** (1) Eye drops (timolol, **pilocarpine,** apraclonidine) to constrict pupil, (2) systemic medications (oral or intravenous [IV] acetazolamide [prevents aqueous humor production], IV mannitol) to widen angle, (3) prostaglandin analogs: latanoprost, travoprost, beta blockers topically, timolol, (4) alpha agonists: clonidine
- **Open Angle:** Treat with (1) topical beta blockers (timolol, betaxolol) to ↓ aqueous humor production

or with pilocarpine to ↑ aqueous outflow; (2) carbonic anhydrase inhibitors, laser trabeculoplasty, or a trabeculectomy can improve aqueous drainage

D. Retinal Detachment

Buzz Words:
- Seeing spots in eyes + no other complaints → retinal detachment
- Sudden vision loss that is sustained + myopic + traumatic injury → retinal detachment

Clinical Presentation: Retinal detachment is the most highly tested acute problem of the eye that will be encountered on the shelf. Look for patients who complain about seeing "spots." Although anyone can have retinal detachment, the likelihood increases with age, and especially occurs in patients with myopia. Other risk factors including diabetes, smoking, glaucoma, acquired immunodeficiency syndrome (AIDS), and pre-eclampsia. Thus, PPx against eye trauma should be maximized in these patients. You will most likely be tested on recognizing the risk factors and the ophthalmologic emergency that detachment presents.

PPx:
- Prevent trauma in myopics, manage diabetes, smoking, glaucoma, AIDS, pre-eclampsia

MoD:
- Retina peels away from rest of eye → vision loss and blindness

Dx:
- Dilated fundoscopic exam

Tx/Mgmt:
1. Retinal reattachment by tilting head back and attaching with surgery, cryotherapy, or injecting expansile gas into eye
2. Scleral buckle: place band around eye to get retina closer to sclera

E. Retinal Vascular Disorders

Buzz Words: Sudden, painless unilateral blindness + cherry red spot on fovea + not hypertensive → central retinal artery occlusion

Rapid, painless vision loss + "blood and thunder" finding on fundoscopic exam + hypertensive → central retinal vein occlusion

Clinical Presentation:

Central retinal artery occlusion: Presents with sudden, painless, unilateral blindness; pupil reacts to near stimulus but is slowly reactive to light; present with

> **QUICK TIPS**
>
> "Curtain" over the eyes = description of vision loss that applies for both retinal detachment and amaurosis fugax. The former is sustained while the latter is transient.

a cherry-red spot on the fovea, retinal swelling, and retinal arteries that may appear bloodless.

Central retinal vein occlusion: Rapid, painless vision loss in a hypertensive; choked, swollen optic disk with hemorrhages; venous stasis retinal hemorrhages; cotton-wool spots; and edema of the macula on fundoscopic exam "Blood and Thunder"

PPx:
- Modifiable risk factors

MoD:
- Occlusion of vascular blood supply either in artery or vein

Dx:
- Fundoscopic exam

Tx/Mgmt:
- **Central retinal artery occlusion:** (1) Intra-arterial thrombolysis of the ophthalmic artery within **8 hours** of onset of symptoms; (2) decrease IOP by draining anterior chamber, ocular massage and high-flow oxygen, IV acetazolamide
- **Central retinal vein occlusion:** (1) Laser photocoagulation

F. Age-Related Macular Degeneration (ARMD)

Buzz Words:
- >50 y/o + gradual painless loss of ventral vision + otherwise normal → dry ARMD
- Diabetic + hypertensive + rapid vision loss + signs of neovascularization on fundoscopic exam → wet ARMD

Clinical Presentation:
- **Atrophic ("dry") macular degeneration:** Responsible for 80% of cases with gradual vision loss
- **Exudative or neovascular ("wet") macular degeneration:** Much less common, but associated with more rapid and severe vision damage.

PPx: (1) Vitamin supplementation, (2) diabetes maintenance, (3) hypertension maintenance

MoD:
- Dry ARMD: Drusen deposition in macula → irreversible damage and vision loss
- Wet ARMD: Abnormal blood vessel growth from vascular endothelial growth factor (VEGF) → bleeding, leaking, irreversible damage

Dx:
- Dry ARMD: (1) fundoscopic exam to look for drusen, pigmented changes
- Wet ARMD: (1) fundoscopic exam to look for hemorrhage and subretinal fluid

Tx/Mgmt:
- Atrophic ARMD: No treatment; vitamin C, E, beta carotene, and zinc supplementation can slow progression.
- Exudative ARMD: (1) VEGF inhibitors (ranibizumab, bevacizumab, pegaptanib) improve vision, slow loss; (2) photodynamic therapy with verteporfin as adjunctive therapy

Infections and Inflammation of the Eye

A. Conjunctivitis
Buzz Words:
- Bilateral watery, discharge, itchy eyes → viral or allergic conjunctivitis
- Unilateral purulent discharge, eyelids stuck together → bacterial conjunctivitis

Clinical Presentation: Rarely directly tested, but frequently seen as a distractor answer choice.

PPx: None

MoD:
- Infection of the eye from bacteria, virus, or from immunogenic allergic response

Dx: Ocular physical exam

Tx/Mgmt:
1. Bacterial form is treated with warm compresses and topical antibiotics.
2. Viral and allergic forms are treated with antihistamines and mast cell stabilizers.

B. Uveitis
Buzz Words:

Photophobia, redness, blurred vision + history of morning back pain → uveitis in the s/o ankylosing spondylitis

Photophobia, redness, blurred vision + aphthous ulcers + genital ulcers → uveitis in s/o Behcet syndrome

Clinical Presentation: Patients with uveitis usually have an underlying medical disorder such as ankylosing spondylitis or Behcet syndrome.

PPx: None

MoD:
- Inflammation of the uvea, failure of the ocular immune system to prevent inflammation and destruction from disease; driven by Th17 cells

Dx:
1. Slit-lamp examination
2. Systemic work-up

Tx/Mgmt: Steroids

> **QUICK TIPS**
>
> Uveitis is associated with systemic disorders such as Behcet syndrome and ankylosing spondylitis.

Traumatic and Mechanical Disorders of the Eye

There are a number of traumatic and mechanical disorders that can happen to the eye, which include burns, abrasions, dislocated lens, and optic nerve injury. The only one that you will be asked to manage is abrasive injury, as the management of other conditions are better reserved for emergency rooms and are out of the scope of the neurology shelf.

A. Corneal Abrasion

Buzz Words: history of trauma + wears contact lens + painful eye + positive fluorescein test

Clinical Presentation: See Buzz Words.

PPx: None

MoD: Dirty contact lens or dirty fingers → scratch cornea

Dx: Fluorescein stain to identify damage to the cornea (Fig. 4.1)

Tx/Mgmt:

1. Supportive
2. Antibiotic management sometimes to prevent conjunctivitis if suspected

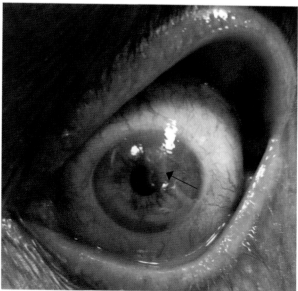

FIG. 4.1 Fluorescein stain. (From Wikimedia Commons: https://commons.wikimedia.org/wiki/File:Human_cornea_with_abrasion_highlighted_by_fluorescein_staining.jpg. Created by James Heilman, MD. Used under Creative Commons Attribution-Share Alike 3.0 Unported license: https://creativecommons.org/licenses/by-sa/3.0/.)

QUICK TIPS

In the shelf, acoustic neuroma always presents in the setting of NF2.

Disorders of the Ear

Although the ear is not a major focus for the neurology shelf, there are a few diseases that are commonly tested: acoustic neuroma, Meniere disease, and benign paroxysmal positional vertigo (BPPV). The difficult part about these is that they all present in a similar way, so be sure to be able to recognize the minutiae that differentiate them. Additionally, they have completely different management processes. The neurology shelf will make a conscious effort to confuse you between these three diseases, so going into this test, be prepared to differentiate the three. If you are pressed for time, don't spend too much time on this section outside of these diseases, although other less commonly tested ear disorders are included here as well.

Primary Disorders of the Ear

A. Acoustic neuroma (neurofibromatosis type II, aka NF2)

Buzz Words: Hearing loss + vertigo + tinnitus + facial pain + café au lait spots → Acoustic neuroma in s/o NF2

Clinical Presentation: See Buzz Words.

PPx: None

MoD: Benign primary intracranial tumor of the myelin-forming cells of the vestibulocochlear nerve (8th cranial nerve). A type of schwannoma, this tumor arises from the Schwann cells responsible for the myelin sheath that helps keep peripheral nerves insulated; NF2 is an inheritable cause of acoustic neuroma

Dx:
1. Physical exam
2. Cranial magnetic resonance imaging (MRI) scan

Tx/Mgmt:
1. Observation
2. Microsurgical removal
3. Radiation

B. Cholesteatoma

Buzz Words:
- Ear discharge and hearing loss with tinnitus, headache, bleeding + abnormal whitish mass seen behind ear drum → cholesteatoma (Fig. 4.2)

Clinical Presentation: Patients with cholesteatoma will always have an abnormal physical exam finding with an otoscopic exam.

PPx: None

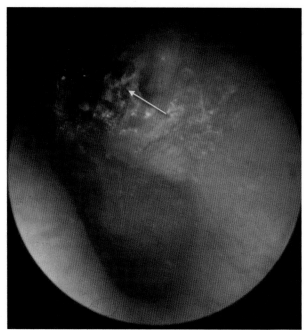

FIG. 4.2 Cholesteatoma. (From Wikimedia Commons: https://commo ns.wikimedia.org/wiki/File:Cholesteatom_kuppelraum_1a.jpg. Created by welleschik. Used under Creative Commons Attribution 2.5 Generic license: https://creativecommons.org/licenses/by/2.5/deed.en.)

MoD: Aberrant growth of keratinizing squamous epithelium in the middle ear and/or mastoid process → expansion into ossicles and spread through skull to brain

Dx: Physical exam with otoscope

Tx/Mgmt: Surgical removal

C. Meniere disease

Buzz Words: Vertigo + tinnitus + hearing loss

Clinical Presentation: Meniere disease is high-yield condition on the shelf given its characteristic triad of vertigo, tinnitus, and unilateral hearing loss. Commonly seen on other shelf exams such as medicine, family medicine, and pediatrics.

PPx: None

MoD: Excess of fluid in inner ear → endolymph bursts from normal channels into other areas

Dx:
1. Clinical history
2. MRI to rule out structural etiologies

Tx/Mgmt:
1. Low-sodium diet
2. Avoid trigger
3. Over-the-counter (OTC) medicine to reduce vomiting
4. Betahistine

D. Benign Paroxysmal Positional Vertigo (BPPV)

Buzz Words: Symptoms of vertigo depending on position of head + nausea and vomiting + no tinnitus

Clinical Presentation: Most common reason for vertigo on the shelf is benign BPPV. Symptoms usually resolve with the Dix-Hallpike maneuver. Make sure to be familiar with exactly what the maneuver is, as sometimes only the motion (rather than the name) of the maneuver is mentioned.

PPx: (1) Avoid triggers (lack of sleep, barometric pressure)

MoD: Calcium crystals are dislodged in inner ear labyrinth → migrate over semicircular canals → displacement

Dx: Dix-Hallpike maneuver

Tx/Mgmt:
1. Dix-Hallpike maneuver
2. Prevent triggers
3. Meclizine, scopolamine

E. Otosclerosis

Buzz Words: Hearing loss over time + family history (FHx) of hearing loss + increased vascularity of promontory seen through the ear drum

Clinical Presentation: Should be on the differential for a patient who presents with hearing loss. More common as a distractor answer choice.

PPx: None

MoD: Overgrowth of bone in middle and inner ear → progressive deafness, etiology unknown

Dx: Clinical findings = Schwartz sign (increased vascularity of the promontory seen through the ear drum)

Tx/Mgmt:
1. Sodium fluoride
2. Surgical treatment

Adverse Drug Effects on the Eye and Ear

Although adverse drug effects on the eye and ear begin to fall out of the scope of the neurology exam, it is important to understand that they exist! There are only a few drugs to know, so better to be safe than sorry in the off chance that any of these are tested. There are two major side effects to know for the eye: Ethambutol is a therapy for tuberculosis, and can cause optic neuritis and a peripheral neuropathy. **Hydroxychloroquine** is a malaria drug and is known to have problems with macular toxicities and retinopathies. There are several drug classes/drugs that have ototoxicity: cisplatin, aminoglycosides, furosemide, and salicylates. The most common manifestation of these is hearing loss.

QUICK TIPS
Vertigo versus Dizziness: Vertigo = "Room is spinning"; Dizziness = "Head is spinning, room is still."

GUNNER PRACTICE

1. A 49-year-old female with no past medical history complains of double vision. Yesterday, she was playing catch with her daughter when a softball hit her in the right eye. She does not remember losing consciousness and has no other complaint other than pain in her right eye, which improves with ibuprofen. Although the conjunctiva on the right eye is red, the fundoscopic examination is normal. When asked to look up, her right pupil remains in the neutral position while her left pupil is elevated. What is the most likely mechanism of this patient's double vision?
   A. Paralysis of cranial nerve VI
   B. Entrapment of superior rectus muscle
   C. Entrapment of superior oblique muscle
   D. Entrapment of inferior oblique muscle
   E. Paralysis of cranial nerve III

2. A 59-year-old man had acute onset of left eye pain, blurred vision, and headache 6 hours ago. He reports no other associated symptoms. On exam, his left eye is nonreactive to light while his right is reactive. There is a noticeable redness in the left conjunctiva and the left eye is bulging out slightly more than the right. Which of the following is the best next step in management of this patient?
   A. Tonometry
   B. MRI of the head and neck
   C. Treatment with timolol
   D. Treatment with carbonic anhydrase inhibitors
   E. Treatment with nonsteroidal antiinflammatory drugs (NSAIDs) for pain relief

3. A 3-year-old boy is brought into the hospital by his mother after she noticed him "wobbling" while walking. She reports nothing else unusual, but did mention that he recently came down with a "cold." On examination, the child is irritable but otherwise alert and oriented. Vital signs were within in normal limits. He has an unsteady gait and is unable to sit upright without support. Cerebrospinal fluid (CSF) analysis shows no red blood cells and Gram stain did not indicate any infectious etiology. What does the child most likely have?
   A. Acoustic neuroma
   B. Benign positional paroxysmal vertigo
   C. Meniere disease
   D. Ataxia-telangiectasia
   E. Acute cerebellar ataxia

Notes

ANSWERS: What Would Gunner Jess/Jim Do?

1. WWGJD? A 49-year-old female with no past medical history complains of double vision. Yesterday, she was playing catch with her daughter when a softball hit her in the right eye. She does not remember losing consciousness and has no other complaint other than pain in her right eye, which improves with ibuprofen. Although the conjunctiva on the right eye is red, the fundoscopic examination is normal. When asked to look up, her right pupil remains in the neutral position while her left pupil is elevated. What is the most likely mechanism of this patient's double vision?

Answer: D, Entrapment of the inferior oblique muscle.

Explanation: Patients who are hit in the eye with some sort of object and can no longer elevate their pupil superiorly classically have inferior oblique entrapment. The mechanism is that the object fractures the orbital floor and the inferior oblique muscle is entrapped in the bone fragments. What makes this question so commonly tested is that the terminology can be tricky since the "inferior" oblique is actually responsible for "superior" movement of the eye. This is a classic scenario that can also appear on the surgery or medicine shelf.

A. Paralysis of cranial nerve VI: Incorrect. Cranial nerve 6 innervates the lateral rectus, which is responsible for lateral motion of the eye. Cranial nerve 6 palsy would present as a patient who complains of diplopia and cannot move his or her pupil laterally past midline.

B. Entrapment of superior rectus muscle: Incorrect. Although the superior rectus is responsible for superior movement of the eyeball, the rectus muscle does not typically get entrapped by a fracture of the superior orbital cavity for two reasons. First, epidemiologically, the fracture is less common for the mechanism of injury. Second, gravity pulls the muscle downward, which makes it less likely to be caught in the bone fragments. In contrast, the inferior oblique muscle is pulled down by gravity toward any potential fracture of the inferior orbital cavity. Although it is possible, for the purposes of the shelf, it is the inferior oblique that is the answer in this type of injury mechanism.

C. Entrapment of superior oblique muscle: Incorrect. This answer may be tempting but it important to keep in mind that the action of the muscle is actually inferior rotation of the eyeball. So entrapment of the superior oblique muscle would lead to an inability to inferiorly, not superiorly, rotate the eyeball.

E. Paralysis of cranial nerve 3: Incorrect. Cranial nerve 3 does not innervate the inferior oblique muscle and would present as a classic "down and out" of the pupil.

2. WWGJD? A 59-year-old man had the acute onset of left eye pain, blurred vision, and headache 6 hours ago. He reports no other associated symptoms. On exam, his left eye nonreactive to light while his right is reactive. There is a noticeable redness in the left conjunctiva and the left eye is bulging out slightly more than the right. Which of the following is the best next step in management of this patient?

Answer: A, Tonometry

Explanation: The acute onset of left eye pain with signs of elevated IOP (e.g., left eye bulging, nonreactive to light) are Buzz Words for closed-angle glaucoma. The first diagnostic step in a patient with suspected closed-angle glaucoma is tonometry. Confirmation of elevated IOP >21 mm Hg necessitates treatment with drugs that constrict the pupil (e.g., timolol). Closed-angle glaucoma is an emergency and is thus frequently tested on the neurology shelf. Onset can be triggered in settings where the pupils dilate, such as being in a dark movie theater.

B. MRI of the head and neck: Incorrect. MRI could be considered if you were concerned about stroke. However, the first diagnostic step for any stroke work-up is a noncontrast head computed tomography (CT) to rule out (r/o) hemorrhage. In this case, the patient's symptoms are more concerning for closed-angle glaucoma than stroke or transient ischemic attack, which would present with temporary complete blindness of one eye.

C. Treatment with timolol: Incorrect. Timolol is often used in treatment of closed-angle glaucoma but is not the correct answer here because the diagnosis needs to be established with tonometry first.

D. Treatment with carbonic anhydrase inhibitors: Incorrect. Although carbonic anhydrase inhibitors can be used as a treatment for closed-angle glaucoma, it is second line. In addition, the diagnosis for this patient had yet to be made.

E. Treatment with NSAIDs for pain relief: Incorrect. Although typically providing someone with immediate pain relief is a reasonable first option, the emergent nature of closed-angle glaucoma requires that the diagnosis and treatment of the underlying cause be made right away.

3. **WWGJD?** A 3-year-old boy is brought in by his mother to the hospital after she noticed him **"wobbling" while walking.** She reports nothing else unusual although and did mention that he **recently came down with a "cold."** She mentions that it makes her dizzy to watch her child walk. On examination, the child is irritable but otherwise alert and oriented. **Vital signs** were within in **normal limits.** He has an unsteady gait and is unable to sit upright without support. **CSF** analysis shows **no red blood cells** and Gram stain did not indicate any **infectious etiology.** What does the child most likely have?

Answer: E, Acute cerebellar ataxia.

Explanation: When you see a young child who presents with ataxia and a recent or ongoing case of infectious illness (viral, bacterial or otherwise), immediately suspect acute cerebellar ataxia. The purpose of this question is to show how ear disorders may be tested on the shelf. While cerebellar ataxia is not an ear disorder per se, its signs and symptoms put ear disorders in the differential. Thus a good understanding of ear disorders (answers A–C) would allow you to rule out enough questions to have a 50–50 shot. The reason why it is not an ear disorder is that the child himself did not complain of any vertigo, tinnitus, or hearing loss. The word "dizzy" is used to describe the mother and is intended as a distractor for those speed-reading the question. Ultimately, acute cerebellar ataxia is the right answer, as it is commonly found in kids with acute illness.

A. Acoustic neuroma: Incorrect. Patient does not have any signs of NF2, which would be present in the question stem if acoustic neuroma were the answer.

B. BPPV: Incorrect. Patient does not report feeling vertigo or dizziness (only the mom reported herself being dizzy). Therefore, this is not BPPV.

C. Meniere disease: Incorrect. Patient does not have tinnitus or any other auditory complaints suggestive of Meniere disease.

D. Ataxia-telangiectasia: Incorrect: Ataxia-telangiectasia is a congenital disorder with symptoms that would be gradual rather than acute.

Cerebrovascular Disease Organizing Principles

Hao-Hua Wu, Leo Wang, and Chuang-Kuo Wu

Cerebrovascular disease is the umbrella term used to describe disease processes in the brain ("cerebro") that are caused by ischemia or hemorrhage ("vascular") because of vascular pathologies of the arterial or venous systems. Stroke, aneurysms, and vascular malformations all fall under the category of cerebrovascular disease. Questions about stroke are high-yield on the Clinical Neurology Shelf because they allow examiners to test multiple organ systems at once. For instance, managing stroke patients with clopidogrel versus warfarin requires understanding of hematology and pharmacology. Aneurysms are also a high-yield topic because of the potential severity of disease. For instance, a subarachnoid hemorrhage (SAH) secondary to a ruptured Berry aneurysm is life threatening, and thus examiners frequently ask for the correct sequence of diagnostic steps needed to rule out a subarachnoid bleed.

There are two organizing principles for this chapter. First, know the anatomy. A total of 50%–65% of questions you will see on this topic will require you to not only diagnose an ischemic or hemorrhagic event, but also localize the lesion and blood supply. Thus, learn the function of each part of the brain (e.g., Wernicke area in the Temporal Lobe → Comprehension of speech) and the topographic layout (e.g., homunculus). Then, master the blood supply to each area of the brain (middle cerebral artery [MCA] → Wernicke area). Once you are familiar with the anatomy, identify the Buzz Words that point to a diagnosis (e.g., No speech comprehension and repetition + Fluent speech = lesion in the Wernicke area). Then learn the mechanism and the prophylactic and treatment measures for the described disease.

Second, divide stroke into either ischemic or hemorrhagic. Each type of stroke has its own Buzz Words and imaging findings. Identifying the kind of stroke in a question stem will enhance the process of elimination.

This chapter is divided into (1) Cerebral Vascular Supply, (2) Ischemic Stroke, (3) Hemorrhagic Stroke, (4) Miscellaneous Neuro Vascular Pathology, and (5) Gunner Practice (application of the material learned). As always,

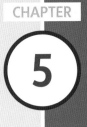

GUNNER COLUMN

QUICK TIPS

3 Steps for Localizing the Lesion
1. ID area of brain dysfunction
2. ID vascular supply
3. ID the mechanism that disrupted the vascular supply (e.g., ischemia vs. bleed)

FOR THE WARDS

Ischemic = 80%
Hemorrhagic = 20%

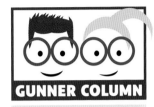

AR
NBME Clinical Neurology Content Outline

each disease process will be divided into the four physician tasks on which the shelf exam will test you: (1) prophylactic management (PPx), (2) mechanism of disease (MoD), (3) diagnostic steps (Dx), and (4) treatment/management (Tx/Mgmt).

Cerebral Vascular Supply

The blood supply to the brain has two arterial origins: (1) the internal carotid arteries (ICAs) left and right (L/R), which supply anterior structures, and (2) the vertebral arteries (L/R), which supply posterior structures. Both the ICAs and vertebrals originate from the aorta, ascend to the brain anteriorly and posteriorly, respectively, branch out, and are linked together by these branches in the Circle of Willis (Fig. 5.1).

A. Anterior circulation

From inferior to superior, the internal carotid artery has five branches: ophthalmic, posterior communicating (PComm), anterior choroidal, anterior cerebral, and the middle cerebral arteries.

1. The ophthalmic artery supplies the retina.
2. The PComm establishes a connection between anterior (internal carotid) and posterior (posterior cerebral artery [PCA]) circulations.
3. The anterior choroidal artery supplies the posterior limb of the internal capsule, and portions of the basal ganglia and thalamus. Lesions of the anterior choroidal artery can lead to isolated contralateral hemiparesis, since the posterior limb of the internal capsule is essential for motor output.
4. The anterior cerebral artery (ACA) supplies the medial frontal and parietal lobes. Also branches into the Heubner artery, which supplies the basal ganglia.

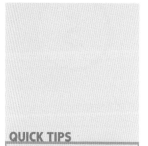
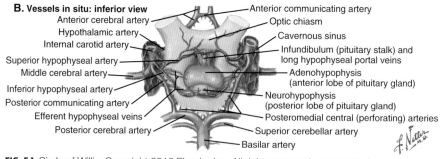

B. Vessels in situ: inferior view
- Anterior cerebral artery
- Hypothalamic artery
- Internal carotid artery
- Superior hypophyseal artery
- Middle cerebral artery
- Inferior hypophyseal artery
- Posterior communicating artery
- Efferent hypophyseal veins
- Posterior cerebral artery
- Anterior communicating artery
- Optic chiasm
- Cavernous sinus
- Infundibulum (pituitary stalk) and long hypophyseal portal veins
- Adenohypophysis (anterior lobe of pituitary gland)
- Neurohypophysis (posterior lobe of pituitary gland)
- Posteromedial central (perforating) arteries
- Superior cerebellar artery
- Basilar artery

FIG. 5.1 Circle of Willis. Copyright 2016 Elsevier Inc. All rights reserved. www.netterimages.com.

5. The middle cerebral artery (MCA) supplies the temporal, lateral frontal, and lateral parietal lobes. The MCA also gives off lenticulostriate arterial branches, which supply the basal ganglia and internal capsule (Fig. 5.2).

B. Posterior circulation

The vertebral arteries are different from the ICAs in that they fuse at the junction between the medulla and pons into the basilar artery. Thus, the posterior circulation for the brain is also known as the vertebrobasilar system.

From inferior to superior, the vertebral artery leads seven arterial structures: (1) anterior spinal artery, (2) posterior inferior cerebellar artery (PICA), (3) basilar artery (technically not a branch but a continuum of both vertebral arteries), (4) anterior inferior cerebellar artery (AICA), (5) superior cerebellar arteries (SCA), (6) PCA, and (7) paramedian arteries to the midbrain and thalamus.

Moreover, the way to organize the penetrating arteries of the vertebral-basilar system is by paramedian versus circumferential arteries. Paramedian arteries (anterior

AR

Cerebral cortex demonstration of cortical structure of the brain

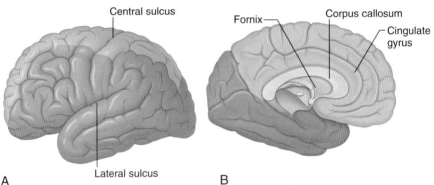

A   B

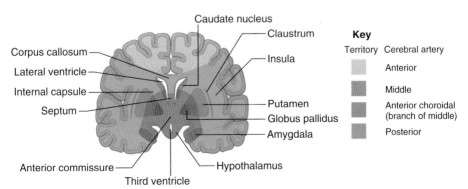

C

FIG. 5.2 ACA, MCA and PCA distributions. **A,** Lateral view of the left cerebral hemisphere. **B,** Saggital view of the left cerebral hemisphere. **C,** Coronal view of the brain through the basal ganglia. From Pentland B: The nervous system. In Naish J, Court DS, editors: *Medical sciences*. 2nd ed. London, 2015, Elsevier Ltd.

spinal arteries, paramedian arteries to midbrain/thalamus) supply midline structures. Circumferential arteries (PICA, AICA, SCA) supply lateral structures.

1. The anterior spinal arteries supply medial brainstem structures, including the corticospinal tract.
2. The PICA supplies lateral medulla, inferior/medial cerebellum, and the choroid plexus of the fourth ventricle.
3. The basilar artery supplies the medial pons directly and lateral pons through the short and long circumferential pontine arterial branches.
4. The AICA supplies the lateral pons, anterior, inferior surface of cerebellum, and middle cerebellar peduncle. AICA also branches off into the internal auditory arteries, which supply the vestibulocochlear nerves into the internal ear.
5. The SCA supplies the superior/lateral aspects of the cerebellum.
6. The PCA supplies the occipital lobe and gives off the thalamoperforator, posterior choroidal, and thalamogeniculate arteries, which supply the thalamus.
7. The paramedian arteries to the midbrain and thalamus supply the medial midbrain and thalamus.

QUICK TIPS

PCA Supplies:
1. Occipital lobe
2. Corpus callosum—splenium

Ischemic Stroke

Organizing Principles for Ischemic Stroke

1. Risk factors (and thus prophylactic measures) are the same for ischemic stroke.
   1. Nonmodifiable risk factors
      - Age = most important risk factor for stroke
      - Men > Women
      - African American > Caucasian
   2. Modifiable risk factors (higher yield)
      - Hypertension (HTN) = most important modifiable risk factor
      - Cardiac disease (e.g., atrial fibrillation [AFib])
      - Diabetes 2/2 increased susceptibility to atherosclerosis
      - Hypercholesterolemia
      - Smoking
      - Drug abuse
      - Coagulopathy
      - Carotid stenosis
      - Homocysteine
2. Anterior versus posterior circulation symptoms
   - Amaurosis fugax → localize to anterior circulation, likely 2/2 internal carotid pathology since ophthalmic artery is involved

QUICK TIPS

The only nonmodifiable risk factor worth remembering is age.

QUICK TIPS

Modifiable risk factors are more high-yield because of potential treatment options. If pressed for time, know HTN, AFib, carotid stenosis.

- Vertigo, dysphagia → localize to posterior circulation, likely 2/2 vertebrobasilar pathology
3. Stroke PPx
    1. Treat hypertension
    2. Statins to treat hyperlipidemia
    3. Aspirin
    4. Tx diabetes
4. MoD: Thrombotic, hypoxic, embolic **(T, H, E)**
    1. **T**hrombotic: Clot forming at site of infarction
    2. **H**ypoxic: 2/2 hypoxemia, hypoperfusion
    3. **E**mbolic: Embolus from distal site travels to brain vasculature
5. Stroke Dx:
    1. Computed tomography (CT) scan
    2. Magnetic resonance imaging (MRI)
    3. Carotid duplex scan → carotid ultrasound)
    4. Echocardiogram to look for cardiac emboli originating in the heart
6. Stroke Tx/Mgmt
    1. If less than 4.5 hours since onset of symptoms (sx) → tissue plasminogen activator (tPA)
    2. Less than 6–8 hours: interventional thrombectomy procedures
    3. Warfarin
    4. Long-term maintenance on antiplatelet agents
    5. Secondary prevention of modifiable risk factors to PPx future strokes
7. Strokes usually, if not always, cause upper motor neuron signs such as Babinski and hyperreflexia (of note, lower motor neuron signs are seen in peripheral nerve diseases and include fasciculations and hyporeflexia).

> **MNEMONIC**
> THE mechanism of ischemic stroke is all the same (Thrombotic, Hypoxic, Embolic).

A. Transient Ischemic Attack (TIA)

Buzz Words: Stroke sx (such as mono-ocular blindness, amaurosis fugax) + <24 hours + no lesions on MRI

Clinical Presentation: On the shelf, TIA most commonly presents as amaurosis fugax with no findings on MRI.

PPx: Manage modifiable risk factors.

MoD: T, H, E of cerebral vasculature, most commonly greater than 80% occlusion of carotid artery

If amaurosis fugax → ICA thrombosis or embolism (anterior circulation)

If vertigo, diplopia → vertebrobasilar insufficiency (e.g., TIA is 2/2 posterior circulation)

Dx:
1. Noncontrast head CT scan to rule out hemorrhagic lesion
2. Brain MRI to verify ischemic lesions

3. Carotid duplex scan or CT angiogram of head/neck or magnetic resonance (MR) angiogram of head/neck → look for extracranial or intracranial stenosis
4. Cardiac Echo (transthoracic echocardiogram [TTE] or transesophageal echocardiography [TEE]) → look for thrombus in left atrium, especially in patients with AFib

Tx/Mgmt: antiplatelet agents or anticoagulation drugs such as
1. Aspirin
2. Clopidogrel
3. Warfarin

B. Carotid Artery Dissection (aka dissection of internal carotid)

Buzz Words: Ptosis and miosis (Horner minus anhydrosis because sympathetic is not on internal carotid) + amaurosis fugax + head and neck pain

Clinical Presentation: Almost exact presentation of vertebral arterial dissection but does not have posterior circulation symptoms

PPx: N/A

MoD: trauma (blunt, penetrating, stretch) → intimal tear → hemorrhage between intima and media of internal carotid → blocks internal carotid lumen → narrower lumen predisposes to thrombosis

Dx:
1. Doppler
2. CT/MRI to rule out (r/o) stroke
3. Helical CT angiogram

Tx/Mgmt:
1. Heparin bridge to warfarin (for at least 3 months)
2. Surgery

C. Vertebral Arterial Dissection

Buzz Words: Head pain + dysphagia, vertigo (postcirculation sx) + Horner syndrome

Clinical Presentation: Almost exact presentation/MoD as carotid dissection, but with posterior circulation symptoms

PPx: N/A

MoD: trauma (blunt, penetrating, stretch) → intimal tear → hemorrhage between intima and media of vertebral artery → blocks internal carotid lumen → narrower lumen predisposes to thrombosis

Dx:
1. Doppler
2. CT/MRI to r/o stroke
3. Helical CT angiogram

Tx/Mgmt:
1. Heparin bridge to warfarin (for at least 3 months)

Ischemic Stroke Pertaining to Anterior Circulation

The two main cerebral vessels of anterior circulation are the MCA and ACA. Both are considered "large vessels," suggesting the MoD is most commonly 2/2 embolism and focal thrombosis leading to stenosis or arterial-to-arterial embolism. Thus, an important theme for MCA, ACA, and PCA strokes is to look for originating emboli in the work-up (w/u). Emboli can originate from the heart, aorta, carotid arteries, and more rarely from amniotic fluid in pregnant women.

Another key about large vessels like the MCA and ACA is that they can be divided into superficial and deep divisions. The superficial divisions supply the cerebrum. The deep divisions supply subcortical structures like the thalamus and basal ganglia.

Finally, due to homunculus organization, the MCA affects the face and upper extremities, whereas the ACA affects the trunk and lower extremities.

A. Large Vessel MCA Stroke

Buzz Words: Upper limb and face paralysis, numbness + contralateral + Wernicke/Broca aphasia (left hemisphere) + hemineglect (right hemisphere) → MCA stroke

Pure motor hemiparesis → stroke affecting lenticulostriate arteries (deep branches of MCA stroke)

Clinical Presentation: MCA stroke is the single most commonly tested ischemic stroke

PPx: Manage modifiable risk factors

MoD: T, H, E of the MCA

If Broca/Wernicke aphasia → MCA stroke on dominant hemisphere (usually left)

If hemineglect → MCA stroke in nondominant hemisphere (usually right)

Dx: Stroke w/u

Tx/Mgmt: Stroke Tx protocol

Types of Aphasia (as seen in stroke syndromes)

"Aphasia": language deficit 2/2 cerebral abnormality
- You should be able to differentiate from "dysarthria," which is language impairment 2/2 cranial nerve or muscular abnormality.

Transcortical: repetition intact, no damage to arcuate fasciculus

Broca aphasia = nonfluent + impaired repetition

Transcortical motor aphasia = nonfluent but intact repetition

Wernicke aphasia = impaired comprehension + impaired repetition

Transcortical sensory aphasia = impaired comprehension but intact repetition

Transcortical mixed aphasia = nonfluent and impaired comprehension with intact repetition

Conduction aphasia = primarily impaired repetition

Global aphasia = nonfluent + impaired repetition + impaired repetition

B. ACA Stroke

Buzz Words: Lower limb paralysis + grasp reflex/behavior abnormalities + transcortical motor aphasia → ACA stroke

Clinical Presentation: Can present with hemiparesis in larger infarcts, which affects lower limbs.

PPx: Manage modifiable risk factors

MoD: T, H, E of the ACA

Dx: Stroke w/u

Tx/Mgmt: Stroke Tx protocol

C. Watershed Infarcts (ACA-MCA border zone or MCA-PCA border zone) (Fig. 5.3)

Buzz Words: Proximal arm weakness/sensory loss + proximal leg weakness/sensory loss + distal extremities OK → watershed infarct of ACA-MCA border

Clinical Presentation: Commonly tested because of unique presentation (paresis of proximal limbs).

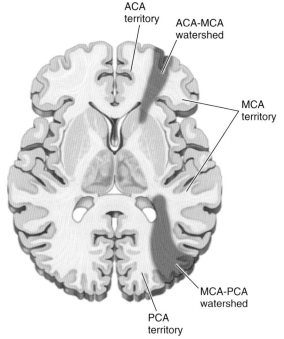

FIG. 5.3 ACA-MCA Watershed area. *ACA,* Anterior cerebral artery; *MCA,* middle cerebral artery; *PCA,* posterior cerebral artery. From Blumenfeld H: *Neuroanatomy through clinical cases.* 2nd ed. Sunderland, MA, 2010, Sinauer Associates, Inc.

PPx: Stroke PPx protocol
MoD: Carotid stenosis, thromboembolism → infarct of water-shed areas (ACA-MCA and MCA-PCA anastomoses)
According to homunculus, proximal arm and legs motor/sensory converge at watershed areas
Dx: Stroke w/u
Tx/Mgmt: Stroke Tx protocol

Lacunar Stroke

Lacunar stroke means stroke of the small vessels of the brain (e.g., the thalamoperforator or lenticulo-striate arteries). Since both anterior and posterior circulation have small vessel branches, lacunar stroke represents a mix of the two. The most common cause of lacunar stroke (as opposed to large-vessel anterior/posterior stroke) is thrombosis from chronic hypertension. Also, unlike large vessel stroke, lacunar stroke often causes distinctive syndromes (i.e., pure motor loss or pure sensory loss). Lacunar stroke is most commonly found in the basal ganglia, thalamus, or basis pontis. Be familiar with Buzz Words and MoD only, because the PPx, Dx, and Tx/Mgmt are similar to the other types of stroke (except with greater emphasis on treating hypertension for prevention).

QUICK TIPS
If motor + sensory, can be MCA/ACA OR a mix of thalamic/internal capsule.

A. Pure Motor Hemiparesis or Dysarthria Hemiparesis
Buzz Words: unilateral face, arm, and leg upper motor neuron (UMN) weakness +/− dysarthria + no other lesions → infarct of posterior limb internal capsule OR ventral pons OR corona radiata OR cerebral peduncle
Clinical Presentation: See Buzz Words.
PPx: Stroke PPx protocol
MoD: There are four possible MoDs:
1. Lenticulostriate artery OR anterior choroidal OR perforating branch of PCA → posterior limb of internal capsule infarct
2. Ventral penetrating branches of basilar artery → small infarction of basis pontis
3. Small MCA branches → corona radiata infarct
4. Small proximal PCA branches → cerebral peduncle infarct
Dx: Stroke w/u
Tx/Mgmt: Stroke Tx

B. Ataxic Hemiparesis
Buzz Words: unilateral face, arm, and leg UMN weakness +/− **ataxia** + no other lesions → infarct of posterior limb

internal capsule OR ventral pons OR corona radiata OR cerebral peduncle

Clinical Presentation: Presents with very mild weakness and ataxia. Also has same MoD as pure motor hemiparesis.

PPx: Stroke PPx protocol

MoD: There are four possible MoDs (same as pure motor hemiparesis)

1. Lenticulostriate artery OR anterior choroidal OR perforating branch of PCA → posterior limb of internal capsule infarct
2. Ventral penetrating branches of basilar artery → ventral pons infarct
3. Small MCA branches → corona radiata infarct
4. Small proximal PCA branches → cerebral peduncle infarct

Dx: Stroke w/u

Tx/Mgmt: Stroke Tx

C. Pure Sensory Stroke (thalamic lacunae)

Buzz Words: Sensory loss (T/P/P) in contralateral face and body + no other focal lesion + sx persist >24 hours → pure sensory stroke 2/2 ventral posterior lateral (VPL) nucleus of thalamus infarct

Clinical Presentation: Be sure to differentiate pure sensory stroke from peripheral nerve pathology. The former typically covers unilateral upper and lower limb; the latter is often isolated to a single limb.

PPx: (1) Stroke PPx protocol

MoD: Thalamoperforator branches of the PCA lesion → VPL nucleus of the thalamus infarct

Dx: Stroke w/u

Tx/Mgmt: Stroke Tx

D. Sensorimotor Stroke (thalamocapsular lacunae)

Buzz Words: Sensory loss (T/P/P) in contralateral face and body + unilateral face and body UMN paresis + sx persist >24 hours + no cerebral involvement → sensorimotor stroke 2/2 VPL and internal capsular infarcts

Clinical Presentation: See Buzz Words

PPx: Stroke PPx protocol

MoD: Thalamoperforator branches of the PCA lesion + lenticulostriate arteries →VPL and posterior limb of internal capsule infarcts

Dx: Stroke w/u

Tx/Mgmt: Stroke Tx

E. Subthalamic lacunar stroke

Buzz Words: Hemiballismus + sx persist >24 hours + no other focal lesions or psych disorder

Clinical Presentation: One of the few disorders in which the patient presents with hemiballismus on the shelf.

PPx: Stroke PPx protocol

MoD: Thrombosis of one of the thalamoperforator arteries

Dx: Stroke w/u

Tx/Mgmt: Stroke Tx

Ischemic Stroke Pertaining to Posterior Circulation

Branches from the PCA and the vertebrobasilar system comprise the posterior circulation of the brain. The easiest way to identify stroke originating from the posterior circulation is to look for cranial nerve signs. For instance, eye movement palsies (CN III, IV, VI), vertigo (CN VIII), dysphagia, dysarthria (CN IX and X), and tongue deviation (CN XII) are symptoms that are easily recognized in question stems. There are more than 10 distinctive brainstem stroke syndromes to remember. The two most common are lateral medullary syndrome (Wallenberg) and paramedian pontine infarct, so they are most likely to come up in clinics. The shelf, however, likes to test the obscure, so make sure to be familiar with the other 13 as well.

A. PCA Stroke

Buzz Words: Homonymous hemianopia (c/l to lesion) + sx >24 hours +/– thalamic aphasia/hemiparesis/sensory loss→ PCA stroke/Homonymous hemianopia (c/l to lesion) + sx > 24 hours + alexia without agraphia (left hemisphere) → PCA stroke involving splenium of corpus callosum

Clinical Presentation: Due to thalamoperforating arteries, PCA stroke can mimic MCA stroke, but is differentiated due to the homonymous hemianopia

PPx: Stroke PPx protocol

MoD: T, H, E.

Dx: Stroke w/u

Tx/Mgmt: Stroke Tx

B. Top of the Basilar Syndrome

Buzz Words: Visual disturbances + memory loss + extraocular movement pathology + ataxia + visual hallucinations (so-called peduncular hallucinosis; put in psych section) + somnolence + delirium → top of the basilar syndrome

Clinical Presentation: See Buzz Words
PPx: Stroke PPx protocol
MoD: Embolus lodges at distal end of basilar artery
　　Visual disturbances 2/2 visual cortex infarct
　　Memory loss 2/2 b/l medial thalami and temporal
　　　lobes
　　Visual disturbances 2/2 CN III infarct of midbrain
　　Ataxia 2/2 cerebellar infarcts
　　Visual hallucinations 2/2 ascending reticular activating
　　　system of midbrain
Dx: Stroke w/u
Tx/Mgmt: Stroke Tx

C. Weber Syndrome (Midbrain Basis)

Buzz Words: Ipsilateral CN III palsy + contralateral hemiparesis infarct + no other focal lesions + sx >24 hours → Weber syndrome 2/2 infarction that damages the CN III nerve and the cerebral peduncle
Clinical Presentation: See Buzz Words
PPx: Stroke PPx protocol
MoD: T, I, E penetrating branches of PCA and/or top of basilar artery → infarct of one side of oculomotor nerve fascicles + cerebral peduncle; as a result, this lesion causes ipsilateral oculomotor palsy and contralateral hemiparalysis
Dx: Stroke w/u
Tx/Mgmt: Stroke Tx

D. Claude Syndrome (Midbrain Tegmentum)

Buzz Words: Ipsilateral CN III palsy + contralateral ataxia + sx >24 hours → Claude syndrome (midbrain tegmentum infarct)
Clinical Presentation: Less commonly tested, but is included in the differential of a CN III palsy
PPx: Stroke PPx protocol
MoD: T, I, E branches of PCA and top of basilar artery → infarct of oculomotor nerve fascicles + superior cerebellar peduncle fibers + red nucleus; sometimes with minimal weakness
Dx: Stroke w/u
Tx/Mgmt: Stroke Tx

E. Benedikt Syndrome (Midbrain Basis and Tegmentum): Combined Weber and Claude syndromes

Buzz Words: Ipsilateral CN III palsy + contralateral ataxia + involuntary tremors + sx >24 hours → Benedikt syndrome

Clinical Presentation: Also less commonly directly tested, but frequently included as a distractor answer choice.

PPx: Stroke PPx protocol

MoD: T, I, E branches of PCA and top of basilar artery → infarct of oculomotor nerve fascicles + superior cerebellar peduncle fibers + cerebral peduncles + red nucleus + substantia nigra infarcts

Dx: Stroke w/u

Tx/Mgmt: Stroke Tx

Mid-Pontine Syndromes

F. Locked-In Syndrome

Buzz Words: Respiratory arrest + no horizontal eye movements + vertical movements intact + whole body paralysis otherwise + bilateral Babinskis

Clinical Presentation: Commonly tested: patient will present as having control of eye movement only.

PPx: Stroke PPx protocol

MoD: T, I, E basilar artery → b/l infarct of the entire ventral portion of pons (so-called basis pontis)

Dx: Stroke w/u

Tx/Mgmt: Stroke Tx

G. Dysarthria Hemiparesis (Pure Motor Hemiparesis 2/2 Paramedian Pontine Infarct)

Buzz Words: Contralateral face and body weakness + dysarthria + no other focal lesions + symptoms >24 hours → dysarthria hemiparesis

Clinical Presentation: Not as high-yield as locked-in syndrome. Dysarthria clumsy hand syndrome is a variant of this disorder. Can also present 2/2 one-side infarction of basis pontis divided at the midline from the other side

PPx: Stroke PPx protocol

MoD: T, I, E paramedian branches of basilar artery/ventral territory → corticospinal tract, corticobulbar tract infarcts

Dx: Stroke w/u

Tx/Mgmt: Stroke Tx

H. Ataxia hemiparesis (2/2 medial basis pontis infarct)

Buzz Words: Contralateral face and body weakness + dysarthria + c/l ataxia → ataxia hemiparesis

Clinical Presentation: Like dysarthria hemiparesis, dysarthria clumsy hand syndrome is a variant of ataxia hemiparesis as well.

PPx: Stroke PPx protocol

MoD: T, I, E paramedian branches of basilar artery/ventral territory → corticospinal tract, corticobulbar tract infarcts + pontine nucleus and pontocerebellar fiber infarcts

Dx: Stroke w/u

Tx/Mgmt: Stroke Tx

Medial Pontine Basis and Tegmentum Syndromes

I. **Foville syndrome (2/2 medial pontine basis and tegmentum)**

Buzz Words: Contralateral face and body weakness + dysarthria + ipsilateral horizontal gaze palsy (CN VI palsy)

Clinical Presentation: Patient chief complaint is typically the CN VI palsy (unable to look laterally).

PPx: Stroke PPx protocol

MoD: T, I, E paramedian branches of basilar artery (ventral/dorsal territory → infarct of superior colliculus, cortico spinal, corticobulbar tracts

Dx: Stroke w/u

Tx/Mgmt: Stroke Tx

J. **Millard Gubler Syndrome**

Buzz Words: Contralateral face and body weakness + dysarthria + ipsilateral facial weakness

Clinical Presentation: Rarely tested directly, but is a distractor answer for patients with CN VII palsy. This disorder is due to a central lesion in the pons

PPx: Stroke PPx protocol

MoD: T, I, E paramedian branches of basilar artery (ventral/dorsal territory → infarct of corticospinal and corticobulbar tracts + the portion of fascicles of facial nerve traveling in the basis pontis.

Dx: Stroke w/u

Tx/Mgmt: Stroke Tx

K. **Pontine Lesions without Names (One-and-a-Half Syndrome)**

Medial lemniscus lesion → contralateral decreased position and vibration 2/2 lesion to paramedian branches of basilar artery (ventral/dorsal territories)

Medial longitudinal fasciculus (MLF) lesion → internuclear ophthalmoplegia (INO) 2/2 lesion to deeper paramedian branches of basilar artery (ventral/dorsal territories)

- Damaging MLF and parapontine reticular formation (PPRF, connects CN VI nucleus and MLF) and one side CN VI nucleus; but sparing the other side CN V1.

- Only one eye can move laterally in a horizontal direction (one-and-a-half paralysis of eye movements)
- The ipsilateral eye (as the "one") cannot move laterally and medially; the contralateral eye (as the "half") cannot move medially but can move laterally because the CN VI is spared)

Lateral Caudal Pons Syndrome

L. AICA Syndrome

Buzz Words: Ipsilateral ataxia + vertigo + nystagmus + loss of pain/temperature (P/T) on ipsilateral face and contralateral body + ipsilateral hearing loss

Clinical Presentation: On the differential for ipsilateral hearing loss. Is differentiated by isolated CN VIII pathology by presence of other symptoms (such as loss of P/T)

PPx: Stroke PPx protocol

MoD: T, I, E AICA, and labyrinthine artery branch → AICA syndrome

Ipsilateral ataxia 2/2 lesion to middle cerebellar peduncle

Vertigo/nystagmus 2/2 vestibular nuclei

Ipsi loss of P/T to face 2/2 trigeminal nucleus/tract

Contra P/T to body 2/2 spinothalamic tract

Ipsilateral hearing loss 2/2 Inner ear

Dx: Stroke w/u

Tx/Mgmt: Stroke Tx

Dorsolateral Rostral Pons Syndromes

M. Superior Cerebellar Artery (SCA) Syndrome

Buzz Words: Ipsilateral ataxia + lesion of SCA territory on MRI

Clinical Presentation: Commonly used as a distractor answer choice with the chief complaint of ipsilateral ataxia.

PPx: Stroke PPx protocol

MoD: T, I, E SCA → infarct of superior cerebellar peduncle and cerebellum → ipsilateral ataxia

Dx: Stroke w/u

Tx/Mgmt: Stroke Tx

N. Medial Medullary Syndrome (Dejerine Syndrome)

Buzz Words: Contralateral body weakness + decreased position/vibration sense + ipsilateral tongue weakness (CN XII palsy)

Clinical Presentation: Commonly tested due to the fact that not many disorders on the shelf cause CN XII palsy

PPx: Stroke PPx protocol

MoD: T, I, E paramedian branches of vertebral and ASA → infarct of pyramidal tract (c/l body weakness) + infarct of medial lemniscus (c/l loss of pos and vib of body) + infarct hypoglossal nucleus (ipsilateral tongue weakness)

Dx: Stroke w/u

Tx/Mgmt: Stroke Tx

O. Lateral Medullary Syndrome (aka Wallenberg Syndrome)

Buzz Words: Ipsilateral ataxia, vertigo, nystagmus, nausea + loss of P/T ipsilateral face and c/l body + ipsilateral Horner syndrome + **hoarseness** and **dysphagia** + ipsilateral decreased taste

Clinical Presentation: One of the most high-yield diseases in this chapter due to diverse presentation. Different from AICA syndrome due to hoarseness and dysphagia since nuclei of cranial nerves IX–XII reside exclusively in the medulla. Because the corticospinal tract (pyramid) is spared, there is no contralateral weakness!

PPx: Stroke PPx protocol

MoD: T, I, E PICA—commonly, cause is due to thrombosis or embolism of PICA → infarct of inferior cerebellar peduncle/vestibular nuclei (ataxia/vertigo/nystagmus/nausea) + infarct of trigem tract (ipsi face loss P/T) + infarct of spinothalamic tract (c/l body loss P/T) + infarct of descending sympathetic fibers (ipsi Horner syndrome) + infarct of nucleus ambiguous (hoarseness/dysphagia) + infarct of nucleus solitaries (ipsi dec taste)

Dx: Stroke w/u

Tx/Mgmt: Stroke Tx

Hemorrhagic Stroke

Hemorrhagic stroke accounts for 20% of all strokes. The following steps are usually taken for PPx and Tx measures:

1. Elevating head of bed above 45 degrees
2. Hyperventilation
3. Acetazolamide

These are the three fastest measures to decrease intracranial pressure (ICP) and blood flow to the head. Make sure to memorize these measures in order, because this is a popular shelf exam topic. This can also be applied for patients with increased ICP due to the swelling effect of ischemic stroke, but will more likely be seen associated with hemorrhagic etiologies.

For the purposes of the shelf, only SAH and venous sinus thrombosis are worth highlighting as a category under hemorrhagic stroke.

Other categories of hemorrhage (traumatic hemorrhage, intracerebral hemorrhage, cerebral artery aneurysm) will be covered in Chapter 9: Traumatic, Mechanical and ICP Disorders in the Neurology Shelf.

A. Subarachnoid Hemorrhage (SAH)

Buzz Words: Worst explosive type headache of life → SAH

Clinical Presentation: Guaranteed to be on your neuro shelf because this disease presents a high risk of mortality, so don't miss it on your clerkship rotation either. Most importantly, remember the work-up (Dx) for SAH as this will undoubtedly save someone's life in the future!

PPx: Decrease blood pressure (BP)

MoD: Rupture of Berry aneurysm

Dx:
1. CT/MRI
2. Lumbar puncture (LP; always consider doing a lumbar puncture if SAH is suspected, but CT/MRI show negative because CT/MRI is only 90% sensitive; LP makes sure you r/o the other 10% of uncertainty)
3. CSF analysis for the evidence of blood (xanthochromic; yellowish)
4. Angiogram to localize the aneurysm that ruptures so that surgical intervention can be planned

Tx/Mgmt:
1. Hemorrhagic treatment protocol
2. Surgery
3. Antihypertensive meds

B. Cerebral Venous Sinus Thrombosis (CVST)

Buzz Words: Headache + seizures + stroke sx (hemiparesis, dysphagia) + patient at thrombotic risk (i.e., hypercoagulable state—postpartum, pregnancy, nephrotic syndrome, polycythemia vera, dehydration in the elderly, etc.; homocystinuria)

Clinical Presentation: High-yield due to association with thrombotic medical comorbidities (e.g., nephrotic syndrome and homocystinuria).

PPx: (1) Blood thinner (e.g., heparin) if recurrent

MoD: Acute thrombosis of dural venous sinuses → no drainage of blood from brain

Dx:
1. CT
2. MRI venogram
3. Cerebral angiography

Tx/Mgmt:
1. Heparin bridge to warfarin,
2. Thrombotomy by interventional procedure if clot still present

C. Superior Sagittal Sinus (SSS) Thrombosis

Buzz Words: Elevated ICP + headache + papilledema + empty delta sign on imaging

Clinical Presentation: SSS thrombosis is a subtype of CVST.

PPx: (1) Blood thinner (e.g., heparin) if recurrent

MoD: acute thrombosis of sagittal sinus → hemorrhagic stroke

Dx:
1. CT
2. MRI venogram
3. Cerebral angiography

Tx/Mgmt:
1. Heparin bridge to warfarin
2. Interventral procedure to remove the thrombus if possible

Miscellaneous Neuro Vascular Pathology

The shelf exam also covers other vascular pathology that is considered neurological but not under the purview of stroke. These disorders are listed below. Make sure to focus on Buzz Words, as Tx/Mgmt is rarely tested.

A. Subclavian Steal Syndrome

Buzz Words: Claudication of arm (coldness, tingling, muscle pain) + visual symptoms + equilibrium problems (posterior neurologic signs) + symptoms in s/o arm exercise

Clinical Presentation: High-yield disorder that is frequently tested on the neurology, medicine, and surgery shelf exams.

PPx: N/A

MoD: Arteriosclerotic stenotic plaque at the origin of the subclavian (before the takeoff of the vertebral) does not allow enough blood supply to reach the arm for normal activity; therefore, the blood pressure would be low on the affected arm. After doing the exercise of the affected arm, the blood flow can be stolen from the ipsilateral vertebral artery (retrograde flow) in order to supply the blood into the brachial artery. As a result, there is not enough blood flow going into the posterior circulation that supplies the brain stem.

Dx:
1. Ultrasound duplex scan
2. Arteriogram (to show reversal of flow of the affected vertebral artery)

Tx/Mgmt:
1. Bypass surgery

B. Vascular Dementia
This will also be covered in the dementia section, but is placed here for emphasis.

Buzz Words: Stepwise decline of cognitive function; memory loss + over the course of disease with history of multiple ischemic or hemorrhagic strokes (weakness, dizziness)

Clinical Presentation: This is often tested in the setting of memory loss as opposed to stroke symptoms.

PPx:
1. Reduce stroke risk factors.

MoD: Thrombosis or embolism of large and/or small arteries

Dx:
1. CT
2. MRI

Tx/Mgmt:
1. Cholinesterase inhibitors
2. Secondary stroke prevention treatments

C. Hypertensive Encephalopathy
Buzz Words: Extensive history (Hx) of severe or malignant hypertension + reversible + headache + papilledema (2/2 hypertension)

Clinical Presentation: Keep a keen eye out for the BP reading; often it is buried within a long question stem.

MoD: (1) Complete blood count (CBC) to r/o microangiopathic hemolytic anemia (MAHA), (2) urinalysis (UA) and basic metabolic panel (BMP) to r/o hypertensive nephropathy, (3) urine drug screening (UDS) to r/o drug-induced hypertensive encephalopathy

Dx:
1. BP measurement (>180/120 with signs of neurologic dmg)
2. MRI

Tx/Mgmt:
1. Nimodipine
2. Labetalol

D. Posterior Reversible Encephalopathy syndrome (PRES; aka Reversible Posterior Leukoencephalopathy Syndrome [RPLS])
Buzz Words: Hypertension (by Hx or physical examination [PEx]) + eclampsia/preeclampsia in s/o pregnancy + headache + seizures + confusion + swelling of brain on neuroimaging + nonreversible

Clinical Presentation: Frequently tested on the ob/gyn shelf as well due to association with eclampsia/preeclampsia, which are disorders of pregnancy associated with high blood pressure.

PPx: (1) Tx HTN

MoD: Can be caused by hypertension, eclampsia

Dx:

1. Measure BP
2. MRI neuroimaging

Tx/Mgmt:

1. BP meds prescribed by family doc/cardiologist

E. Brain Arteriovenous Malformations (ARMs)

Buzz Words: Severe headache + seizure + hemorrhage w/o history of trauma + clump of vessels seen on neuroimaging

Clinical Presentation: AVMs are abnormal connections between arteries and veins that bypass capillaries. It most commonly presents as hemorrhage 2/2 AVM rupture.

PPx: None

MoD: Unknown

Dx:

1. CT to detect bleeding
2. MRI w/contrast to visualize AVM

Tx/Mgmt:

1. Surgery, if possible

F. Ectasia of Cerebral Vessels

Buzz Words: Cranial nerve deficit + bulge of cerebral vessels seen on CT/MR angiogram → ectasia of cerebral vessels

Clinical Presentation: Ectasia means distension. Vessel ectasia means a blood vessel has distended and is causing symptoms by adjacent compression. It can also be described in the term "dolichoectasia," which means elongation and compression. Ectasia most commonly affects the vertebral or basilar arteries. For example, the compression to the CN V can cause trigeminal neuralgia.

PPx: (1) Tx hypertension

MoD: Deterioration of tunica intima/media of the blood vessel → distension → compresses neighboring structures/nerves

Dx:

1. Angiogram

Tx/Mgmt:

1. Surgery

GUNNER PRACTICE

1. A 71-year-old man comes to the hospital 2 hours after a brief episode of left arm weakness, which has since resolved. He denies losing consciousness and has never had symptoms like this before. The patient takes metformin for diabetes mellitus and lisinopril for hypertension. He retired from his job as a teacher 6 years ago and denies tobacco or alcohol use. His vitals are 151/93 mm Hg, 99.3 F, 70 bpm, 14 RR, and PaO_2 96% on room air. The exam is notable for a carotid bruit that is heard on the right, and is otherwise normal. Troponin and CK-MB are within normal limits. An electrocardiogram shows a normal sinus rhythm, and echocardiography shows no structural abnormalities. An 85% right internal carotid stenosis is discovered on carotid duplex ultrasonography. What is the best prophylactic measure to prevent cerebral infarction?
   A. Metoprolol
   B. Simvastatin
   C. Surgical removal of carotid artery plaque
   D. Exercise regimen and low-sodium diet
   E. Warfarin

2. A 74-year-old man is brought to the emergency room after a 9-hour history of word-finding difficulty and weakness in the right arm and leg. His past medical history is notable for diabetes type 2, hypertension, hyperlipidemia, and atrial fibrillation. Current medications include aspirin, atorvastatin, lisinopril, and hydrochlorothiazide. He is alert and oriented but has trouble answering your questions. His vitals are 184/94 mm Hg, 98.7F, 84/min, and 20/min. There is weakness and decreased sensation in the right upper and lower extremities with a Babinski sign present only on the right side. Which of the following is the most appropriate next step in diagnosis?
   A. Carotid duplex ultrasonography
   B. Echocardiography
   C. A noncontrast head CT
   D. Lumbar puncture
   E. Cerebral angiography
   F. Electroencephalography

3. A 72-year-old woman comes to the physician complaining of dizziness and lightheadedness for the past 3 weeks. Her medical history is notable for hypertension, for which she is taking hydrochlorothiazide, lisinopril, and a beta-blocker. When she rises from a seated

position, she feels light-headed and takes several minutes to collect herself. Her blood pressure is 120/80 mm Hg in the right arm and 70/35 mm Hg in the left arm while she is lying down; upon standing, her blood pressure is 85/55 mm Hg in the right arm and 60/35 mm Hg in the left arm. Her physical exam is unremarkable. Carotid ultrasonography shows reverse flow in the right vertebral artery with no signs of occlusion. What is the appropriate next step in management?

A. Coronary arteriography
B. Adjust her medication regimen
C. Transesophageal echocardiography
D. Prophylactic warfarin
E. Carotid endarterectomy

Notes

ANSWERS: What Would Gunner Jess/Jim Do?

1. WWGJD? A 71-year-old man comes to the hospital 2 hours after a brief episode of left arm weakness, which has since resolved. He denied losing consciousness and has never had symptoms like this before. The patient takes metformin for diabetes mellitus and lisinopril for hypertension. He retired from his job as a teacher six years-ago and denies tobacco or alcohol use. His vitals are 151/93 mmHg, 99.3F, 70 bpm, 14 RR, and PaO2 96% on room air. The exam is notable for a carotid bruit is heard on the right, and is otherwise normal. Troponin and CK-MB are within normal limits. An electrocardiogram shows a normal sinus rhythm, and echocardiography shows no structural abnormalities. An 85% right internal carotid stenosis is discovered on carotid duplex ultrasonography. What is the best prophylactic measure to prevent cerebral infarction?

Answer: C, Surgical removal of carotid artery plaque

Explanation: The patient has TIA likely 2/2 a clot thrown off by ICA stenosis. Carotid stenosis that are ≥80% is an indication for carotid endarterectomy, which is a procedure that removes the plaque from the carotid artery. It is important in this question not to become caught up in the filler between the first and second-to-last sentence, because the degree of stenosis makes C the best answer.

A. Metoprolol → Incorrect. The patient's hypertension is a risk factor for stroke and likely contributed to the ICA stenosis. However, controlling the BP with metoprolol is not as effective a prophylactic measure as carotid endarterectomy if the stenosis is ≥80%.

B. Simvastatin → Incorrect. There are two quick ways to rule out this answer. First, there is no mention of hyperlipidemia so there is no need to treat. Second, the MoD was 2/2 carotid stenosis and given the risk of stroke in the near future, a more drastic measure is needed than a long-term medication.

D. Exercise regimen and low-sodium diet → Incorrect. While it is likely the patient will benefit from an exercise regimen and low-sodium diet, it is also not as effective of a prophylactic measure given the degree of stenosis.

E. Warfarin → Incorrect. Warfarin is used in s/o AFib and deep vein thrombosis (DVT) to prevent emboli formation and release. If one does not see cardiac disease, warfarin is unlikely to be the answer when it comes to management of stroke.

2. WWGJD? A 74-year-old man is brought to the emergency room after a 9-hour history of word-finding difficulty and weakness in the right arm and leg. His past medical history is notable for diabetes type 2, hypertension, hyperlipidemia and atrial fibrillation. Current medications include aspirin, atorvastatin, lisinopril, and hydrochlorothiazide. He is alert and oriented but has trouble answering your questions. His vitals are 184/94 mmHg, 98.7F, 84/min, and 20/min. There is weakness and decreased sensation in the right upper and lower extremities with a Babinski sign present only on the right side. Which of the following is the most appropriate next step in diagnosis?

Answer: C, Head CT to rule out hemorrhagic stroke

Explanation: This is a classical presentation of thromboembolic stroke. This man has both word-finding difficulty indicating Broca aphasia and weakness indicating dysfunction to descending motor tracts. He has all the risk factors (hypertension, hyperlipidemia, diabetes) and even has atrial fibrillation as a potential mechanism for a thromboembolism. His exam further corroborates this diagnosis, demonstrating sensory loss in addition to motor weakness and a Babinski sign, which is only found in upper motor neuron lesions.

A. Carotid duplex ultrasonography → Incorrect. Only indicated if there were suspicion of interruption to blood flow via the carotids; such occlusions would not present so acutely.

B. Echocardiography → Incorrect. Although this may assist in a better understanding of the mechanism of stroke, this is not necessary at this time because this person has already undergone a cerebral infarction.

D. Lumbar puncture → Incorrect. Only indicated if he had symptoms suggesting meningitis, which would include fever, stiff neck, and confusion.

E. Cerebral angiography → Incorrect. Although this would aid in diagnosis, it is really only used for suspected vascular malformations. Although this may occur later if cases prove to be complicated, the first step in managing a stroke acutely is a head CT.

F. EEG → Incorrect. Only indicated for seizures, and nothing suggests seizures here.

3. WWGJD? A 72-year-old woman comes to the physician complaining of dizziness and lightheadedness for the past 3 weeks. Her medical history is notable for hypertension, for which she is taking hydrochlorothiazide, lisinopril, and a beta blocker. When she rises from a seated position, she feels light-headed and takes several minutes to collect herself. Her blood pressure is 120/80 mm Hg in the right arm and 70/35 mm Hg in the left arm while she is lying down; upon standing, her blood pressure is 85/55 mm Hg in the right arm and 60/35 mm Hg in the left arm. Carotid ultrasonography shows reverse flow in the right vertebral artery with no signs of occlusion. What is the appropriate next step in management?

Answer: B, Adjust her medication regimen

Explanation: Although this patient is presenting with clear indication of subclavian steal, she is asymptomatic (subclavian steal will typically cause neurologic symptoms in the affected arm). A bigger problem she is having is orthostatic hypotension, which is the result of her taking three blood pressure medications: hydrochlorothiazide, lisinopril, and a beta blocker. This is causing her to have dizziness and lightheadedness. Thus, adjusting her medication regimen is most important for the next step in management.

A. Coronary arteriography → Incorrect. There is nothing to suggest a blockage or aneurysm in her head.

C. Transesophageal echocardiography → Although it is possible that she has some underlying heart condition that leads to her hypotension, it is more likely that she has orthostatic hypertension secondary to her medications.

D. Prophylactic Warfarin → Incorrect. Warfarin would be indicated in a patient at a high risk for thromboembolism. There is nothing in this patient to suggest this action would be warranted, especially in the absence of any cardiac or cerebral infarction history.

E. Carotid Endarterectomy → Incorrect. Carotid endarterectomy is done to prevent stroke. Before such a procedure would be indicated, she would need a carotid ultrasound, which would tell you if there is a blockage. There is nothing in this patient to suggest that.

Notes

Infections of the Central Nervous System

Leo Wang, Hao-Hua Wu, and Chuang-Kuo Wu

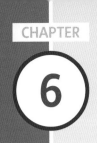

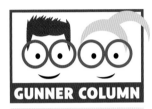

The most high-yield topic in this chapter is meningitis, which is the most frequently tested infection of the central nervous system (CNS). The second most commonly tested topic is Creutzfeldt-Jakob disease (CJD; i.e., "mad cow disease"). If you need to save time, peruse the sections on meningitis, learn the buzz words for CJD, and skip directly to Gunner Practice. Other infectious disorders, such as the ones that cause subacute/chronic encephalitis, are required topics but appear less frequently.

Acute Meningitis

The most common infection you will be tested on is acute bacterial meningitis. Remembering the causes of meningitis by age group is extremely important, as it dictates which treatment modality you choose. For instance, Group B Strep is the single most important cause of bacterial meningitis in infants (0–6 months), because it naturally colonizes the mother's vagina, leading to infection. Second, recognize that *Escherichia coli* and other gram-negative rods (which naturally colonize the gastrointestinal [GI] tract) and Listeria (a food-borne disease) chiefly cause meningitis in infants and the elderly, who are susceptible to fecal-oral spread of these bacteria due to weakened immune systems. Finally, recognize that *Streptococcus pneumoniae*, *Neisseria meningitidis*, and *Hemophilus influenzae* are natural colonizers of the nasopharynx and oropharynx, and thus the most common causes in everyone else. *N. meningitidis* is spread by close contact, and is therefore the most important cause in college students, who spend lots of time in dormitories. *S. pneumoniae* overall is the most common cause of meningitis because of its prevalence in the nasopharynx. Occasionally, meningitis can occur from invasive procedures like neurosurgery—in these situations, be wary of bacteria that live in skin flora, such as staph and MRSA.

Treatment is even easier to remember. Ampicillin covers Listeria and vancomycin covers MRSA. Third generation cephalosporins cover all other causes of bacterial meningitis.

QUICK TIPS

Ampicillin = Listeria.

A. Acute Bacterial Meningitis

Buzz Words: Headache + fever + meningismus + photophobia + altered mental status + seizures + Kernig sign + Brudzinski sign → acute meningitis
- Petechiae + maculopapular rash → *N. meningitidis*
- Unimmunized child → *H. influenzae*

Clinical Presentation: Acute bacterial meningitis is commonly tested and identified if Kernig and Brudzinskis sign are positive. Kernig sign is when passive extension of the knee from flexed, supine position elicits pain. Brudzinski sign is elicited if flexion of the neck results in spontaneous flexion of the hips.

PPx:
1. Vaccines against *N. meningitidis* and *H. influenzae* type B (HiB) for children and compromised adults
2. Exposed contacts in *N. meningitidis* receive PPx with ceftriaxone, rifampin, or ciprofloxacin

MoD:
- Causes:
  - Neonates (<6 months): GBS > GNRs (*E. coli*) > *Listeria monocytogenes*
  - Children (6 months–6 years): *S. pneumoniae* > *N. meningitidis* > *H. influenzae*
  - Adults (6–60 years): *S. pneumoniae* > *N. meningitidis*
  - Elders (>60 years): *S. pneumoniae* > GNRs (*E. coli*) > *Listeria monocytogenes*
  - Invasive CNS processes: *S. aureus* and coagulase negative staph species
- Bacteria from feces or skin → nasal cavity → meninges → infection and inflammation
  - Most common in children and adults
- Bacteria from bloodstream → meninges → infection and inflammation
  - More common in infants and elderly
- Can lead to thrombophlebitis (venous thrombosis in cortical veins and sinuses)
  - Look for CN palsies and diplopia

Dx:
1. Lumbar puncture
   - Increased opening pressure, increased polymorphonucleocytes (PMNs), increased protein, decreased glucose

2. CSF and blood culture
3. Computed tomography (CT) before low pressure (LP) if there is any suspicion for bleeding (papilledema, trauma, immunosuppression, focal findings)
   - In these patients, LP creates negative pressure in CSF → brain herniation
4. Magnetic resonance imaging (MRI)/electroencephalogram (EEG)

Tx/Mgmt:
1. Dexamethasone first to decrease inflammation → prevents neurologic sequelae
2. Antibiotic regimen by age group
   - Infants: ampicillin, third-generation cephalosporin
   - Immunocompromised: third-generation cephalosporin, vancomycin
   - Everyone else: third-generation cephalosporin, vancomycin, ampicillin
3. Supportive: analgesics, antipyretics, antiemetics
4. Anticoagulation with heparin, as needed for deep vein thrombosis (DVT) PPx

B. Acute Viral Meningitis (Aseptic Meningitis)

Buzz Words:
- Summertime; exanthema; hand, foot, and mouth disease (coxsackievirus); herpangina; pleurodynia → echovirus aseptic meningitis
- Mollaret-like PMNs → West Nile virus meningitis

Clinical Presentation: Acute viral meningitis is chiefly caused by three types of viruses: enteroviruses, arboviruses, and herpesviruses. Arboviruses and certain types of herpesviruses also tend to present with encephalitis, which is an infection of the brain parenchyma (meningoencephalitis). You can easily tell the difference between meningitis and meningoencephalitis, because encephalitis almost always causes altered consciousness. Recognize the three viral causes of meningitis and also which specifically cause encephalitis, as well. Enteroviruses are the most common cause of viral meningitis, and most cases occur during the summer. In adults, herpes simplex virus (HSV) can also cause meningitis. Generally speaking, viral meningitis is less common than bacterial meningitis.

PPx: Polio vaccine

MoD:
- Causes
  - Enteroviruses: poliovirus, coxsackievirus, echovirus
    - Most common cause of viral meningitis

- Herpesviruses: HHV1 (HSV1), HHV2 (HSV2), HHV3 (VZV), HHV4 (EBV), HHV5 (CMV)
  - HSV1, HHV3, HHV4 cause meningoencephalitis
- Arboviruses: LaCrosse, West Nile, St. Louis, eastern equine encephalitis virus, western equine encephalitis virus
  - All cause meningoencephalitis
- HIV
- Viral infection outside of brain → hematogenous spread → meninges
- Feces → nasal cavity → meninges → infection and inflammation
  - Poliovirus
- Retrograde spread along peripheral nerves → meninges
  - Herpesvirus

Dx:
1. LP
   - Normal/high opening pressure, increased lymphocytes, increased/normal protein, normal sugar
   - Xanthochromia (RBCs in CSF) from HSV meningoencephalitis
2. CSF/blood culture with CSF PCR
3. Magnetic resonance imaging (MRI)/CT/EEG

Tx/Mgmt:
1. Acyclovir
2. Ganciclovir/foscarnet for suspected CMV
3. Supportive: analgesics, antipyretics, antiemetics

C. Acute Amebic Meningitis

Buzz Words: Altered mental status and meningitis signs after swimming in lake, pond, hot spring, pond, neti pots

Clinical Presentation: Amebic meningitis is rare but deadly, which means it is fair game for the shelf. Luckily, they both present the same way and have no treatment. There are two important causes, acanthamoeba and naegleria fowleri, both of which cause a meningoencephalitis.

PPx: None; avoid swimming in a pond or river that contains ameba.

MoD: Acanthamoeba or *Naegleria fowleri* in freshwater → nasal tissue → olfactory nerve tissue → cribriform plate → meninges

Dx:
1. LP/MRI/CT/EEG
2. CSF wet mount for *N. fowleri*

Tx/Mgmt:
1. Supportive; contact CDC for an investigational drug treatment

QUICK TIPS
LP of bacterial vs. viral meningitis; bacterial = PMNs vs. viral = no PMNs and many lymphocytes.

D. Acute Eosinophilic Meningitis

Buzz Words: Food consumption, Asia, Hawaii, Caesar salad, LP with eosinophilia

Clinical Presentation: Rarely, you may be tested on eosinophilic meningitis, which is characterized by high eosinophilic content in the CSF. The majority is caused by a parasitic nematode, *Angiostrongylus cantonensis*. Patients are infected by ingesting larvae, which can penetrate the GI tract and make its way to the meninges through hematogenous spread. Most cases are self-limited.

PPx: None

MoD: Ingestion of larvae from *Angiostrongylus cantonensis, Baylisascaris procyonis, Gnathostoma spinigerum, Strongyloides stercoralis* → GI tract penetration → hematogeneous spread → meninges

Dx:

1. LP with culture

Tx/Mgmt:

1. Supportive

E. Lyme Neuroborreliosis (2/2 Lyme disease)

Buzz Words: Hiking in woods + erythema migrans + fever + muscle aches + altered mental status → Neuroborreliosis 2/2 Lyme disease

Clinical Presentation: Lyme disease is very high-yield for the shelf. Patients present with a targetoid rash (erythema migrans) and can be treated by doxycycline over the age of 8.

PPx:

1. Minimize exposed skin during hikes.

MoD: Tick bite → infection by Borrelia species → bloodstream → meninges

Dx:

1. Physical exam
2. LP + MRI/CT

Tx/Mgmt:

1. Doxycycline
2. Third generation cephalosporins

Subacute Meningitis

When meningitis presents for longer than 2 weeks, it is considered subacute and warrants further investigation. Any causes of subacute meningitis can also cause chronic meningitis if it lasts longer than 1 month. The causes of subacute meningitis are not as obvious, as they include tuberculosis, fungi, and syphilis. Any of the causes of chronic meningitis, listed later, can also cause subacute meningitis as well.

A. Subacute Tubercular Meningitis

Buzz Words: Headache + stiff neck + fever + lethargy for days to weeks + risk factors for tuberculosis

Clinical Presentation: Be on the lookout for patients who get meningitis in the setting of TB risk factors, such as prior imprisonment and travel to a TB endemic country.

PPx: PPx against tuberculosis (PPD, isoniazid, BCG vaccine)

MoD: Primary *Mycobacterium tuberculosis* infection from droplet inhalation → CNS → caseating tubercles in the brain

Dx:

1. PPD
2. LP with culture

Tx/Mgmt:

1. Rifampin, isoniazid, pyrazinamide, ethambutol

B. Subacute Fungal Meningitis

Buzz Words:

Signs of pulmonary infection (e.g., productive cough) +

- Spelunking + Ohio valley → histoplasmosis
- Southwestern United States + Mexico + Central America → coccidiomycosis
- Acquired immunodeficiency syndrome (AIDS) → Cryptococcus

Clinical Presentation: Most cases of fungal infections are self-limited and don't even cause meningitis. When they do, you might expect that your patient is immunocompromised. Know that these infections start in the lungs, so look for pulmonary symptoms. To determine the etiology, use the patient's location to guide you. Histoplasmosis predominates in the Ohio valley, while Coccidiomycosis will predominate in the California/New Mexico region. Cryptococcus is an opportunistic organism that likes to infect immunocompromised hosts such as elderly diabetes mellitus or HIV patients with a CD4 count less than 100/μL. Use these clues to help you when you suspect a fungal meningitis.

PPx: Cryptococcal antigen screening in AIDS with CD4 <100 cells/μL

MoD: Inhalation of spores from *Cryptococcus* sp., *Histoplasma capsulatum, Coccidia* sp. → pulmonary infection → hematogenous spread → meninges

Dx:
1. LP (Cryptococcal antigen in LP; Eosinophilia in coccidiomycosis)
2. India ink for Cryptococcus

Tx/Mgmt:
1. Cryptococcus: amphotericin B, flucytosine
2. Histoplasmosis, coccidiomycosis: amphotericin B

C. Subacute Syphilitic Meningitis (Neurosyphilis)

Buzz Words: Argyll-Robertson pupil + ataxia + neuropathies + dementia + Romberg sign + neurogenic bladder + hydrocephalus + Charcot joint

Clinical Presentation: Syphilitic meningitis is only a minor complication of untreated infection by Treponema pallidum; the other complications are worse. In the context of untreated syphilis, look for things besides meningitis. Tabes dorsalis, Argyll Robertson pupil, and other neurogenic deficits tend to be more clinically characteristic of tertiary syphilis than anything else.

PPx: None

MoD: Untreated syphilis → meningitis after 1–2 years with hydrocephalus → potential stroke → paresis (10 years) with declining function → tabes dorsalis (20 years)

Dx:
1. LP
2. VDRL, FTA-AB with clinical features
3. MRI/EEG

Tx/Mgmt:
1. Penicillin G

Chronic Meningitis

Chronic meningitis (>1 month) or meningoencephalitis causes include the same causative organisms in subacute meningitis, including syphilis and tuberculosis, but include a few new names. While these organisms are certainly important, they are not as frequently tested as the causes of acute bacterial and viral meningitides. Also recognize that while the majority of acute meningitides are infectious in nature, many of the chronic meningitides are not. Therefore maintain a high level of suspicion of other noninfectious causes when you approach these types of questions.

A. Chronic Bacterial Meningitis

Buzz Words:
- Liver damage + kidney failure + bleeding → Weil disease 2/2 leptospirosis

- Evidence of meningismus for >4 weeks → chronic bacterial meningitis

Clinical Presentation: Chronic bacterial meningitis is caused by species you are less likely to have heard of in the context of neurology (and are thus less likely to be tested on!). Nevertheless, it is important at the very least to recognize their names. You will not be asked how these infections are treated.

PPx: None

MoD:

- Brucella, Actinomycosis, Nocardiosis, Leptospirosis → chronic infection of the meninges

Dx:

1. LP with CSF culture
2. CT/MRI showing dural enhancement
3. Electrophysiologic testing
4. Meningeal biopsy

Tx/Mgmt:

1. Varies by etiology

Encephalitis

Acute Encephalitis

Acute encephalitis is by definition viral; the etiologies for the acute encephalitides are the same as those of acute viral meningitides that are discussed on p. 92.

Subacute/Chronic Encephalitis

There are only two causes of chronic encephalitis, and both are related to something you get from a single measles, mumps, rubella (MMR) vaccine. The only difference is that subacute sclerosing panencephalitis (SSPE) is caused by an untreated measles infection, while progressive rubella panencephalitis (PRP) is caused by congenital rubella contracted from the mother. Use this to differentiate between the two. Although both can be very easily prevented, they are fatal if contracted with no existing cure.

A. Subacute Sclerosing Panencephalitis (SSPE)

Buzz Words: No vaccination + mood and personality changes + headache and seizures + myoclonus + ataxia + quadriplegia + spasticity

Clinical Presentation: High-yield for both the neurology and pediatric shelf, because it is associated with measles and seen in patients who have risk factors for being unvaccinated.

PPx: Vaccine against measles
MoD: Replication of untreated measles virus in neurons and glial cells → progressive neurodegenerative disease
Dx:
1. LP, measles antibodies
2. MRI increased T2 signal
3. EEG: nonspecific slowing, high voltage sharp slow waves of 3–8 seconds
Tx/Mgmt:
1. Detected early, immunomodulators and antivirals
2. Detected late, supportive therapy

B. Progressive Rubella Panencephalitis (PRP)
Buzz Words: Congenital rubella syndrome (deafness, eye abnormalities, congenital heart disease)
PPx: Vaccine against rubella
MoD: Congenital rubella syndrome → latent period of 8–19 years → replication in neurons
Dx:
1. LP → CSF: lymphocytic pleocytosis, rubella oligoclonal bands
2. MRI/EEG
Tx/Mgmt:
1. Supportive

Cerebritis (Abscess)

Cerebritis is by definition the formation of an abscess, a site of inflammation, and collection of infected material due to an infectious source. An abscess can occur either in the cerebrum or the epidural space.

A. Cerebral Abscess
Buzz Words: Otitis media + mastoiditis + sinusitis + pyogenic infection + penetrating trauma + neurosurgery + elevated ICP (papilledema) → cerebral abscess
Ring enhancing lesion on imaging + AIDS → Toxoplasma gondii
Clinical Presentation: Cerebral abscesses form when bacteria infect the brain parenchyma and causes focal weakening, leading to necrosis and a capsulate abscess to wall off the infection. Importantly, the causes of cerebral abscess are different in healthy versus immunocompromised individuals.
PPx: None
MoD: Bacterial infection of brain parenchyma from contiguous, hematogenous or cryptogenic site → coagu-

lative necrosis and abscess capsulate formation →
ring-enhancing with necrotic center
Dx:
1. MRI > CT, ring enhancement of abscess capsule
Tx/Mgmt:
1. Antimicrobial therapy depending on causative organism
2. Anticonvulsant therapy as PPx for seizures
3. Neurosurgical drainage
4. Brain biopsy to rule out lymphoma if no response to
antimicrobials

B. Epidural Abscess
Buzz Words: Fever + headache + seizures with periorbital
edema and frontal bone osteomyelitis + limb weakness
from radiculopathy
Clinical Presentation: You will rarely be tested on an epidural
abscess, but when you do it will almost always present
in the context of a complication from osteomyelitis,
especially in the frontal bone. Look for evidence of
neurologic dysfunction with periorbital edema.
PPx: None
MoD: Spread from osteomyelitis → infection of epidural
space
Dx:
1. MRI
2. LP with CSF culture
Tx/Mgmt:
1. Antibiotic therapy, supportive

Other Infections of the Nervous System
Nontoxin Mediated
A. Poliomyelitis
Buzz Words: Missed vaccinations + paralysis + areflexia +
meningitis
Clinical Presentation: Typically present as a pediatric patient
who has some form of paralysis and has limited history
of vaccination
PPx: Several doses of polio vaccine
MoD: Infected feces → mouth → intestinal mucosa →
replicates within GI cells → hematogenous spread to
meninges → rarely paralytic polio from spinal polio or
bulbar polio or both → weakness, loss of reflexes,
flaccid paralysis

Dx:
1. LP with elevated lymphocytes and polioantibodies
2. Stool sample/pharynx swab → poliovirus culture
Tx/Mgmt:
1. Supportive

B. Creutzfeldt-Jakob Disease (CJD)

Buzz Words: Myoclonic jerks with rapidly altered mental
    status + memory impairment + triphasic spikes on EEG
    ("burst" EEG)

Clinical Presentation: CJD is a commonly tested topic on
    the neuro shelf because it mimics diseases that cause
    memory impairment and seizures. The distinguishing
    factor is the triphasic spikes on EEG. Make sure to
    know that CJD is mediated by a protein (prions).

PPx: Avoid infected human or animal tissue

MoD: Mechanisms include prion protein caused by spo-
    radic (unknown etiology), familial (mutated protein),
    or iatrogenic (tissue infection from someone else)
    mechanisms → misfolding of proteins in neurons
    causing misfolding of other proteins

Dx:
1. LP: 14-3-3 protein and Tau
2. MRI: DWI/T2-FLAIR signal changes in caudate and
    putamen and cortical ribbon sign
3. EEG: periodic sharp wave complex
Tx/Mgmt:
1. Supportive

C. Neurocysticercosis

Buzz Words: Convulsion + CT/MRI findings + cystic lesions
    involving cerebral cortices

Clinical Presentation: This infection is caused by the
    tapeworm—Taenia solium—that resides in pork.
    In the United States, most cases are reported in
    the southern states. Commonly neurocysticercosis
    causes epilepsy, which leads to the diagnosis in
    these patients.

PPx: Avoid contaminated food

MoD: Uncooked pork that contains tapeworm and
    cysticerci → penetrating intestinal wall—hematogenic
    pathway—CNS parenchyma

Dx:
1. Serology (blood EITB) better than CSF (ELISA)
2. CT/MRI showing cystic lesion
3. EEG
4. Lesion biopsy

Tx/Mgmt:
1. Albendazole, praziquantel
2. Steroid for brain edema

Toxin Mediated

A. Botulism

Buzz Words: Honey + floppy baby
Clinical Presentation: Make sure to differentiate from polio, which would typically present much later. Also, ingestion or exposure to honey is classic for botulism.
PPx: Avoid honey for babies.
MoD: Bacterial spores of *C. botulinum* → botulism toxin in blood → nerves → inhibits release of acetylcholine via SNARE proteins → muscle weakness in cranial nerves
Dx:
1. Test stool or enema with bioassay, clinical mostly
Tx/Mgmt:
1. Botulinum antitoxin

B. Tetanus

Buzz Words: Rusty nail injury + muscle spasms + spasms in facial muscle (Risus sardonicus)
Clinical Presentation: Commonly tested on the shelf, especially with regard to MoD
PPx: Immunization with tetanus toxin
MoD: Infection with tetanus toxin → retrograde transport → prevents inhibitory motor neurons from secreting GABA → lockjaw
Dx:
1. Wound bacterial cultures
2. Spatula test: touch posterior pharyngeal wall, and look for either jaw contraction or gag reflex
Tx/Mgmt:
1. Tetanus shot
2. Tetanus IG

GUNNER PRACTICE

1. A 65-year-old man presents to the hospital with a complaint of severe pain in his chest for the past 3 days. He has no significant past medical or family history. The pain is constant and does not get better or worse with activity. The patient's cardiovascular exam is age-appropriate. On inspection, there is a 5-cm vesicular, sharply bordered erythema across T5 on the right side

of the thorax. What is the most appropriate treatment for this patient's disease?

A. Oral acyclovir
B. Intravenous acyclovir
C. Nitrates
D. Oral oseltamivir
E. Intravenous oseltamivir

2. A 41-year-old man with HIV is brought to the hospital by his caretaker concerning odd behavior for a week. The patient caretaker says he has become unusually sedentary to the point where he no longer goes to buy groceries or gets things to eat. He has also been noncompliant with his medications. On exam, patient has swollen lymph nodes, global hyperreflexia, and positive Babinski sign bilaterally. Labs show a CD4 <100. A CT scan of the head shows ring enhancement after contrast administration to an area of the basal ganglia and frontal lobe. What is the most likely organism to cause this patient's symptoms?

A. Herpes simplex
B. Pneumocystis jirovecii
C. Echinococcus
D. Cryptococcus
E. Toxoplasma gondii

3. A 19-year-old college freshman is brought to the hospital by her roommate. The patient reports an aversion to light, headache, and fever, which all began 5 hours ago. Her blood pressure is 120/80, with a pulse of 105/min and temperature of 101°F (38.3°C). Her exam is notable for reddish lesions on her upper and lower extremities, as well as nuchal rigidity. Which of the following is the next best step in the management of the roommate who has been in contact with the patient?

A. Oseltamivir
B. Rifampin PPx
C. Doxycycline PPx
D. Lumbar puncture of the roommate
E. Rifampin if symptoms appear

Notes

ANSWERS: What Would Gunner Jess/Jim Do?

1. **WWGJD?** A 65-year-old man presents to the hospital with a complaint of severe pain in his chest for the past 3 days. He has no significant past medical or family history. The pain is constant and does not get better or worse with activity. The patient's cardiovascular exam is age-appropriate. On inspection, there is a 5-cm vesicular, sharply bordered erythema across T5 on the right side of the thorax that was painful upon palpation. What is the most appropriate treatment for this patient's disease?

   Answer: B, intravenous acyclovir.

   Explanation: The answer to this question requires two steps. First, it is necessary to identify this disease as herpes zoster. This can be straightforward with the physical exam findings. If you see a vesicular painful rash in an older individual that is suggested to be in a dermatomal distribution, then suspect zoster. The second component is treatment, which is a little trickier. Answer choice C should be immediately eliminated as this is clearly a dermatologic/neurologic rather than a cardiovascular issue. That leaves us with PO or IV acyclovir versus PO or IV oseltamivir. This requires you to have a basic familiarity with drug names. The suffix "vir" suggests that they both target viruses. Oseltamivir targets the influenza strains and is used strictly (at least for the purposes of the shelf) for flu patients. So D and E are eliminated. Finally with A and B, one needs to keep in mind the practical difference to oral versus intravenous medication. Oral meds means the patient is going home, while IV means that the patient needs to stay longer. Given the severity of the pain, patients are typically given IV acyclovir for treatment of zoster. Thus, pick B and feel confident about it.

   A. Oral acyclovir → Incorrect. While acyclovir is the treatment for HSV, it is likely that this patient requires inpatient treatment (e.g., intravenous) for relief of symptoms.

   C. Nitrates → Incorrect. Taken for cardiac related chest pain. In this case, the dermatomal findings make a cardiac etiology for the pain much less likely.

   D. Oral oseltamivir → Incorrect. Oseltamivir is used to treat influenza.

   E. Intravenous oseltamivir → Incorrect. Oseltamivir is used to treat influenza.

2. **WWGJD?** A 41-year-old man with HIV is brought to the hospital by his caretaker concerning odd behavior for a week. The patient caretaker says he has become

unusually sedentary to the point where he no longer goes to buy groceries or gets things to eat. He has also been noncompliant with his medications. On exam, patient has swollen lymph nodes, global hyperreflexia and positive Babinski sign bilaterally. Labs show a CD4 <100. A CT scan of the head shows ring enhancement after contrast administration to an area of the basal ganglia and frontal lobe. What is the most likely organism to cause this patient's symptoms?

Answer: E, *Toxoplasma gondii*

Explanation: Typically the buzzword for Toxoplasma is a patient with cats, as toxo can be transmitted through cat litter. However, another common presentation is an AIDS patient (as inferred here by CD4 <200) with multiple ring enhancing solid lesions. Herpes simplex will present as lesions of the temporal lobe, ruling out A. *Pneumocystis jiroveci* does not have a characteristic CT finding, which makes B less likely. Echinococcus would present with space occupying cysts, which is not described in this question stem. And Cryptococcus has nonspecific neurologic findings. That leaves E, toxoplasma, as the best answer choice for this question.

A. Herpes simplex → Incorrect. Classic sign for HSV encephalitis is signal in the bilateral medial temporal lobes on MR1.

B. *Pneumocystis jiroveci* → Incorrect. Pneumocystis does not have a characteristic CT finding.

C. Echinococcus → Incorrect. Would present with space occupying cysts instead of a ring-enhancing lesion.

D. Cryptococcus → Incorrect. Unlikely to cause neurologic findings as seen in this question stem.

3. WWGJD? A 19-year-old college freshman is brought to the hospital by her roommate. The patient reports an aversion to light, headache and fever, which all began five hours ago. Her blood pressure is 120/80, pulse of 105/min and temperature of 101°F (38.3°C). Her exam is notable for reddish lesions on her upper and lower extremities as well as nuchal rigidity. Which of the following is the next best step in the management of the roommate who has been in contact with the patient.

Answer: B, Rifampin PPx

Explanation: Rifampin is the antibiotic of choice for PPx against Neisseria meningitis, which is the most common cause of meningitis for young adults. The classic clinical scenario is a young college patient who presents nuchal rigidity, petechiae, and photophobia. There have been several stories in the news over the past 5 years reporting college students who have died from this type of meningitis. There is both a vaccine and antibiotic PPx that can be provided. Doxycycline is not used as a PPx for meningitis. Oseltamivir is only used for influenza treatment. Lumbar puncture would not be necessary for the roommate, unless she displayed symptoms of meningitis. Also, it is not wise to wait until symptoms arise to take rifampin; given the rapid progression of the disease, waiting for symptoms to appear before taking treatment may be fatal.

A. Oseltamivir → Incorrect. Influenza medication; not used for meningitis PPx.

C. Doxycycline PPx → Incorrect. Not used for meningitis PPx.

D. Lumbar puncture of the roommate → Incorrect. No need for an invasive procedure unless roommates starts exhibiting symptoms.

E. Rifampin if symptoms appear → Incorrect. Rifampin is to prevent symptoms from appearing in the first place and would not be effective if symptoms were already presenting.

Neoplasms of the Nervous System

CHAPTER

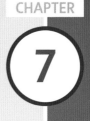

7

George Hung, Hao-Hua Wu, Leo Wang, and Chuang-Kuo Wu

Neoplasms of the nervous system are rare but potentially deadly. Be sure to divide them into benign and malignant types. Compared to Step 1, central nervous system (CNS) tumors appear less on the shelf exam. Also, histology is *NOT* tested, so there is no need to remember things like psammoma bodies or Horner-Wright rosettes (and if you still remember the associated neoplasms then you are a *TRUE* gunner). The most common tumor tested is craniopharyngioma. Nevertheless, be familiar with the neoplasms indicated on the USMLE Content outline and know the key stem clues. Also, remember that neoplasms can occur in the brain, spine, and peripheral nervous system.

The most common tumors in the CNS are cerebral metastases. The most common tumors in adults are supratentorial: glioblastoma multiforme (GBM), meningioma, and schwannoma. The most common tumors in children are infratentorial: pilocytic astrocytoma, ependymoma, and medulloblastoma. The CNS tumor that is most likely to metastasize is the medulloblastoma.

CNS tumors commonly present with progressive ("crescendo") focal neurological deficit, raised intracranial pressure (ICP), seizures, hydrocephalus, and endocrine disturbances. In general, CNS tumors are diagnosed via neuroimaging studies and biopsy. Tumors may manifest as ring-enhancing parenchymal mass lesions, but keep in mind the differential diagnosis includes cerebral abscess, toxoplasmosis, radiation necrosis, resolving hematoma, stroke, trauma, demyelinating lesions, and so on. General treatment principles for CNS tumors include steroid (dexamethasone) for edema, tumor removal, and chemotherapy.

Finally, an organizing principle for neoplasms is that the location of the tumor can cause symptoms based on the function the structures that it compresses. Thus one can use the principles learned in the cerebrovascular chapter to ascertain how a patient would present given tumor location (Fig. 7.1). For instance, a "temporal lobe glioma" may

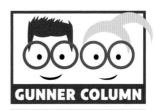

GUNNER COLUMN

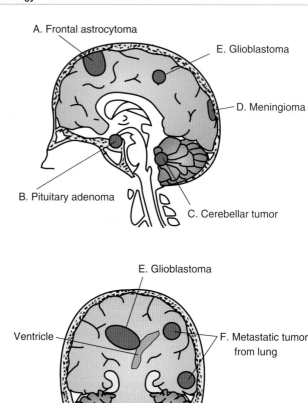

A. Frontal astrocytoma

E. Glioblastoma

D. Meningioma

B. Pituitary adenoma

C. Cerebellar tumor

E. Glioblastoma

Ventricle

F. Metastatic tumor from lung

FIG. 7.1 Effects of brain tumors in various locations. **A** and **D,** Tumors on surface of brain. **B,** Pituitary tumor causes neurologic dysfunction and hormonal abnormalities. **C,** Cerebellar tumors, even when small, can interfere with vital brain stem function. **E,** Tumors in the interior of the brain shift ventricles and interfere with the flow of cerebrospinal fluid. **F,** Multiple metastasis. (From Gould B, Dyer R: *Pathophysiology for the health professions.* St Louis, 2011, Saunders. Fig. 5.12.)

gg AR

MRI/CT images

MNEMONIC

Benign Tumors
　PAPAC MeHN 12 = Pituitary Adenoma, Pilocytic Astrocytoma, Craniopharyngioma, Meningioma, Hemangioblastoma, Neurofibromatosis 1 and 2
　Malignant Tumors
　GOMEM = Glioblastoma Multiforme, Oligodendroglioma, Medulloblastoma, Ependymoma, Metastatic
　Craniopharyngioma = CCR = Children, Calcification, Rathke pouch
　Pituitary Adenoma = P for Prolactinoma

lead to Wernicke aphasia or memory disturbances since the temporal lobe affects both functions.

If you are pressed for time, this is a chapter you can skim or just do the questions for. The most high yield diseases here are neurofibromatosis I and II, as well as craniopharyngioma.

Benign Neoplasms of the Nervous System

Benign neoplasms are the most frequently tested in this chapter. Know the Buzz Words and clinical presentation, and be familiar with the diagnostic steps, although primarily diagnosis is made through biopsy and imaging.

A. Meningioma
Buzz Words:
- Occipital headache + slurred speech + atrophy/fasciculation of tongue + weakness in b/l body + Babinski sign b/l + "streak"/"tail" (dural attachment) seen on magnetic resonance imaging (MRI) → Meningioma of the foramen magnum

Clinical Presentation: Meningioma is one of the most common brain tumors in the pediatric population. For the shelf, you do not need to know the histology. It is oftentimes asymptomatic in real life, but will likely present on the shelf with symptoms

PPx: Reduce ionizing radiation

MoD: Arises from arachnoid cells of the meninges
- Extraaxial

Dx:
1. MRI
2. Biopsy

Tx/Mgmt:
1. Resection
2. Radiation

B. Neurofibromatosis I (aka von Recklinghausen disease)
Buzz Words: Optic nerve glioma + café au lait spots + iris hamartomas (Lisch nodules) + pheochromocytoma + dermal neurofibromas

Clinical Presentation: Neurofibromatosis I (NFI) is one of the most high-yield diseases in this chapter. It is easily recognizable with its combination of café au lait spots and Lisch nodules. It is likely to be tested on the neuro, medicine, pediatrics, and surgery shelf.

PPx: None

MoD: Tumor arises from neural crest cells (don't have to memorize for shelf; learn for own interest only).
- 2/2 mutation of neurofibromin on chromosome 17, a tumor suppressor gene and downregulator of RAS

Dx:
1. Head computed tomography (CT)
2. Urine metanephrines to Dx pheochromocytoma

Tx/Mgmt:
1. Surgery

C. Neurofibromatosis II (aka vestibular schwannomas)
Buzz Words:
- Hearing loss + tinnitus + dizziness + schwannoma + enlarged internal auditory canal extending into cerebellopontine angle → Vestibular schwannomas
- Bilateral vestibular schwannoma → NF2

NF 1 Symptoms

Clinical Presentation: Bilateral vestibular schwannomas is NF2 until proven otherwise

PPx: None

MoD: Arises from Schwann cells, most typically in CN8

Dx:

1. CT

Tx/Mgmt:

1. Surgery
2. Radiation

D. Craniopharyngioma

Buzz Words: Bilateral temporal hemianopsia (aka no peripheral vision OR traffic accident because patient didn't see oncoming car) + calcifications in Rathke pouch + headaches + urinary frequency + children

Clinical Presentation: This diagnosis should be considered whenever the patient presents with temporal hemianopsia. Calcifications in Rathke pouch are also pathognomonic.

PPx: None

MoD: Tumor cells from remnants of Rathke pouch
- Tumor compresses medial side of optic tract at chiasm leading to b/l hemianopsia
- Urinary frequency 2/2 posterior pituitary compression (no antidiuretic hormone [ADH])

Dx:

1. Head CT, MRI

Tx/Mgmt:

1. Surgery
2. Radiation

E. Pituitary adenoma

Buzz Words: Bilateral temporal hemianopsia (aka no peripheral vision OR traffic accident because patient didn't see oncoming car) + prolactinoma + other overactive/ underactive pituitary conditions

Clinical Presentation: Pituitary adenoma is similar to craniopharyngioma but has pituitary side effects and no calcifications in Rathke pouch.

PPx: None

MoD: (Don't have to memorize for shelf.) Tumor cells from pituitary cells (can be any of them)
- Tumor compresses medial side of optic tract at chiasm leading to b/l hemianopsia

Dx:

1. Head CT, MRI

Tx/Mgmt:

1. Surgery
2. Radiation

F. Pilocytic Astrocytoma

Buzz Words: Seizures + cystic appearance on imaging and gross exam + posterior fossa (e.g., cerebellum) + GFAP positive + children

Clinical Presentation: Pilocytic astrocytoma is the most common posterior fossa tumor in children. It may appear on answer choice as simply "astrocytoma."

PPx: Reduce ionizing radiation

MoD: Arises from astrocytes; a subtype of astrocytoma (Grade I)

Dx:
1. Head CT/MRI
2. Biopsy

Tx/Mgmt:
1. Surgery

G. Hemangioblastoma

Buzz Words: Retinal angiomas (associated with von Hippel-Lindau [VHL] syndrome) + secondary polycythemia (erythropoietin production) + family history of renal cell carcinoma + well-circumscribed cyst in cerebellum (most common), spinal cord, or other dural-based location

Clinical Presentation: For the purposes of the shelf, hemangioblastoma of the CNS is von Hippel-Lindau disease until proven otherwise.

PPx: None

MoD: Vascular/stromal origin, mutation in VHL tumor suppressor gene

Dx:
1. Gadolinium-enhanced MRI

Tx/Mgmt:
1. Surgery (gross total resection)
2. Radiation therapy for recurrent or residual disease

QUICK TIPS

Prolactinoma is most common finding from pituitary adenoma; look for galactorrhea.

Von Hippel-Lindau (VHL) disease

Malignant Neoplasms of the Nervous System

Malignant neoplasms are less commonly tested because the shelf focuses primarily on treatable diseases. However, it is good to be aware of these diseases, as they may come up as distractor answer choices. GBM is the most commonly tested malignant nervous system neoplasm because of its characteristic butterfly shape on imaging.

Of note, the USMLE content outline states that astrocytomas are one topic to be familiar with. Astrocytomas are a diverse group of tumors, and the most commonly tested astrocytoma types are GBM and pilocytic astrocytoma. The latter is considered benign.

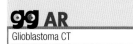

Glioblastoma CT

A. Glioblastoma multiforme (GBM)

Buzz Words: Butterfly lesion on CT + personality changes + located in cerebral hemispheres + adult + GFAP positive astrocyte stain

Clinical Presentation: GBM is one of the most frequently tested tumors because of its characteristic butterfly lesion on CT. Many questions on the shelf will expect you to diagnose GBM based solely on the CT scan, so make sure you know the characteristic lesion well.

PPx: None

MoD: Arises from astrocytes, a subtype of astrocytoma (grade IV)

Dx:
1. Head CT/MRI
2. Biopsy

Tx/Mgmt:
1. Surgery
2. Chemotherapy
3. Radiotherapy

B. Medulloblastoma

Buzz Words: Cerebellar location + Ataxia + children + hydro-cephalus + drop metastases to spinal cord

Clinical Presentation: Medulloblastoma is seen in children and puts the patient at risk for drop metastases in the spinal cord. The most common chief complaint is ataxia.

PPx: None

MoD: Arises from primitive neuroectodermal cells, making it a type of primitive neuroectodermal tumor (PNET)

Dx:
1. Head CT/MRI
2. Biopsy

Tx/Mgmt:
1. Radiotherapy
2. Surgery
3. Chemotherapy

C. Oligodendroglioma

Buzz Words: Frontal lobe tumor + seizure + calcified mass lesion + slow growing + seizures

Clinical Presentation: Rarely tested but frequently used as a distractor answer.

PPx: None

MoD: Arises from oligodendrocytes

Dx:
1. Head CT/MRI
2. Biopsy

Tx/Mgmt:
1. Radiotherapy
2. Surgery
3. Chemotherapy

D. Ependymoma
Buzz Words: Fourth ventricle tumor + hydrocephalus + children
Clinical Presentation: Rarely tested but frequently used as a distractor answer.
PPx: None
MoD: Arises from ependymal cells of the fourth ventricle
Dx:
1. Head CT/MRI
2. Biopsy
Tx/Mgmt:
1. Surgery

E. Metastatic tumors
Buzz Words: Multiple ring-enhancing lesions at the gray-white junction
Clinical Presentation: Patient presentation depends on the location of the metastases. When there are multiple ring enhancing lesions at the gray-white junction, automatically suspect metastasis and try to deduce the primary.
PPx: Reduce ionizing radiation
MoD: Lung cancer, breast cancer, skin cancer, kidney cancer, or colon cancer metastases
Dx:
1. CT/MRI
2. Rule out other etiologies (e.g., neurocysticercosis) with cerebrospinal fluid (CSF) examination, chest X-ray, abdomen ultrasound, body CT scan, and so on
3. Confirmation with biopsy
Tx/Mgmt:
1. Biopsy
2. Surgery
3. Radiation

GUNNER PRACTICE

1. A previously healthy 12-year-old girl is brought to the physician by her mother because of a 1-month history of severe daily headaches and blurred vision. Menarche has not yet begun. She is at the 23rd percentile for height and 69th percentile for weight. Vital signs are

within normal limits. Examination shows bitemporal visual field defects, papilledema, and bilateral weakness of eye abduction. A large suprasellar mass containing numerous specks of calcium is seen on CT scan. Which of the following is the most likely diagnosis?

A. Craniopharyngioma
B. Idiopathic intracranial hypertension (HTN)
C. Medulloblastoma
D. Migraine
E. Parasagittal meningioma
F. Pituitary adenoma
G. Subdural hematoma
H. Temporal lobe glioma

2. A 61-year-old man complains of 6 months of progressive difficulty walking and tripping over his own shoes. He has had a frontal headache for the past 4 weeks. On physical exam, he has spasticity in the legs and hyperactive reflexes with bilateral extensor plantar reflexes. Otherwise, his sensory and strength exams are normal. What does he most likely have?

A. Craniopharyngioma
B. Idiopathic intracranial HTN
C. Medulloblastoma
D. Migraine
E. Parasagittal meningioma
F. Pituitary adenoma
G. Subdural hematoma
H. Temporal lobe glioma

3. An 18-year-old woman comes into the emergency department complaining of morning headaches and nausea and becomes increasingly unsteady on her feet. She says that these symptoms have gradually gotten worse over the past month. Her vital signs are within normal limits. On exam, she has papilledema, mild left facial weakness, and decreased ability to perform the finger-to-nose test with her left limb. What is the most likely diagnosis?

A. Craniopharyngioma
B. Idiopathic intracranial HTN
C. Medulloblastoma
D. Migraine
E. Parasagittal meningioma
F. Pituitary adenoma
G. Subdural hematoma
H. Temporal lobe glioma

Notes

ANSWERS: What Would Gunner Jess/Jim Do?

1. WWGJD? A previously healthy 12 year-old girl is brought to the physician by her mother because of a 1-month history of severe daily headaches and blurred vision. Menarche has not yet begun. She is at the 23rd percentile for height and 69th percentile for weight. Vital signs are within normal limits. Examination shows **bitemporal visual field defects, papilledema, and bilateral weakness of eye abduction. A large suprasellar mass containing numerous specks of calcium is seen on CT scan. Which of the following is the most likely diagnosis?**

Answer: A, Craniopharyngioma

Explanation: This question is a classic craniopharyngioma question stem because it indicates "bitemporal visual defects" (bilateral hemianopsia) and calcification of Rathke pouch (e.g., "suprasellar mass...specks of calcium"). Thus one can immediately select craniopharyngioma based on those Buzz Words. The one answer choice that may serve as a distractor is pituitary adenoma. However, since this patient does not have any pituitary signs/symptoms, one can ascertain that the tumor is not arising from the pituitary.

B. Idiopathic intracranial HTN → Incorrect. Patients with IIH (aka pseudotumor cerebri) present with headache and papilledema, but do not have a mass on neuroimaging (hence the word "idiopathic" in its name). Thus B is ruled out.

C. Medulloblastoma → Incorrect. Medulloblastomas typically occur in kids and can present as a headache (i.e., sx of hydrocephalus). However, they are located in the cerebellum, and thus can be ruled out as an answer choice.

D. Migraine → Incorrect. Migraines are common causes of headache that can present with associated visual symptoms. However, they are not associated with intracranial masses, and are instead 2/2 sensitization of cerebral artery nerve endings.

E. Parasagittal meningioma → Incorrect. Meningiomas are derived from arachnoid cells of the meninges and are thus extraaxial. The fact that the calcifications were suprasellar in the question stem rules out parasagittal meningioma.

F. Pituitary adenoma → Incorrect. Pituitary adenomas are the hardest to differentiate from craniopharyngiomas because both present with bilateral hemianopsia. However, pituitary adenomas have signs and symptoms indicating overproduction of pituitary hormones. Thus, although this patient's "urinary frequency" can be potentially traced back to dysfunction of the posterior pituitary, this is due to deficiency of ADH rather than overproduction of ADH. Pituitary adenoma of the posterior pituitary would lead to no urination and hyponatremia, since ADH would fill up the collecting tube with aquaporins. Thus this answer choice is incorrect. Other common presentations of pituitary adenoma, especially for a girl, would be expression of milk from mammillary nipples 2/2 prolactinoma.

G. Subdural hematoma → Incorrect. Unlikely since there is no mention of bleeding on the neuroimaging report. If the question stem does not directly state it, assume it isn't there.

H. Temporal lobe glioma → Incorrect. No temporal symptoms, such as Wernicke aphasia or memory loss is present in this patient. Thus a glioma in the location of the temporal lobe is unlikely.

2. WWGJD? A 61-year-old man complains of 6 months of progressive difficulty walking and tripping over his own shoes. He has had a frontal headache for the past 4 weeks. On physical exam, he has spasticity in the legs and hyperactive reflexes with bilateral extensor plantar reflexes. Otherwise, his sensory and strength exams are normal. What does he most likely have?

Answer: E, Parasagittal meningioma

Explanation: This patient's leg spasticity, hyperactive reflexes, and bilateral Babinski's indicate a bilateral upper motor neuron (UMN) lesion to the legs. His difficulty walking and tripping are not cerebellar processes, but rather manifestations of UMN lesions to the pathways relating to his legs. A parasagittal meningioma is the most likely, especially in light of the frontal location of his headache. The parasagittal location of this tumor causes bilateral UMN deficits in the region of both the left and right motor homunculi corresponding to the lower extremities.

A. Craniopharyngioma → Incorrect. There are no visual field deficits, and the patient is likely too old to be presenting with a craniopharyngioma.

B. Idiopathic intracranial HTN → Incorrect. Patients with IIH do present with headache, but this patient does not present with papilledema, cranial nerve deficits, or other signs of increased ICP.

C. Medulloblastoma → Incorrect. Although this patient's incoordination and headache may be a signs of cerebellar dysfunction and hydrocephalus, respectively, medulloblastomas typically manifest in children. In addition, it is less likely for a medulloblastoma to cause UMN signs.

D. Migraine → Incorrect. Migraines are common causes of headache that can present with associated visual symptoms. However, they are usually unilateral with associated nausea, photophobia, or phonophobia, and do not manifest with UMN signs.

F. Pituitary adenoma → Incorrect. Patient shows no signs or symptoms indicating overactive or underactive pituitary hormone secretion.

G. Subdural hematoma → Incorrect. Unlikely due to the extended time course (6 months), and lack of head trauma.

H. Temporal lobe glioma → Incorrect. No temporal symptoms, such as Wernicke aphasia or memory loss, are present in this patient. Thus a glioma in the location of the temporal lobe is unlikely.

3. WWGJD? An 18-year-old woman comes into the emergency department complaining of morning headaches and nausea and becomes increasingly unsteady on her feet. She says that these symptoms have gradually gotten worse over the past month. Her vital signs are within normal limits. On exam, she has papilledema, mild left facial weakness, and decreased ability to perform the finger-to-nose test with her left limb. What is the most likely diagnosis?

Answer: C, Medulloblastoma

Explanation: Medulloblastoma is most commonly a cerebellar tumor, which can lead to gait ataxia. It can compress the fourth ventricle, leading to hydrocephalus and symptoms of increased ICP, such as headaches, nausea, and papilledema, as well as cranial nerve deficits, such as facial weakness.

A. Craniopharyngioma → Incorrect. There are no visual field deficits.

B. Idiopathic intracranial HTN → Incorrect. Although the patient does show signs of increased ICP, the cause of increased ICP is not idiopathic. IIH would not cause isolated left limb dysmetria; it is the medulloblastoma that would cause both left limb dysmetria and increased ICP.

D. Migraine → Incorrect. Migraines are common causes of headache and nausea that can present with associated visual symptoms. However, they are usually unilateral with associated photophobia or phonophobia, and do not manifest with isolated left limb dysmetria or papilledema.

E. Parasagittal meningioma → Incorrect. Meningiomas are derived from arachnoid cells of the meninges and are thus extraaxial. The fact that there is left limb dysmetria points to a cerebellar lesion, which is infratentorial.

F. Pituitary adenoma → Incorrect. Unlikely due to lack of visual field deficits, and no indication of overactive or underactive pituitary hormone secretion.

G. Subdural hematoma → Incorrect. Unlikely due to lack of head trauma.

H. Temporal lobe glioma → Incorrect. No temporal symptoms, such as Wernicke aphasia or memory loss is present in this patient. Thus a glioma in the location of the temporal lobe is unlikely.

Spine and Spinal Cord Disorders in the Neurology Shelf

Hao-Hua Wu, Leo Wang, and Chuang-Kuo Wu

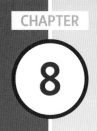

GUNNER COLUMN

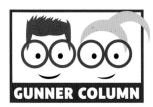

As mentioned in Chapter 2, the spinal cord is another part of the central nervous system (CNS); it is more associated with the peripheral nervous system (PNS) than the brain. The spine is the vertebral column that surrounds and protects the spinal cord. If you get one take-home point from this page, remember that *spine* and *spinal cord* refer to two very different things.

This section is organized into (1) "Disorders of the Spine" and (2) "Disorders of the Spinal Cord." In "Disorders of the Spine," you will learn about issues that deal directly with bone and cartilage, such as spinal stenosis (narrowing of the vertebral canal), disc herniation (bulging of the intervertebral disc out of its normal place), and vertebral osteomyelitis (infection of the bone). Memorize the Buzz Words and the diagnostic steps for these, but most importantly, know how to differentiate benign from emergent pathology. Emergent disorders include infection, malignancy, and cauda equina syndrome (which is covered in the next section), and thus are frequently tested.

In the "Disorders of the Spinal Cord" section, remember the difference between cauda equina and conus medullaris. Also, remember the significance of seeing both upper motor neuron (UMN) and lower motor neuron (LMN) signs simultaneously but at different levels (spinal cord compression). These disorders are frequently tested, so make sure to learn the Buzz Words well.

Disorders of the Spine (Vertebral Column)

This section pertains only to musculoskeletal diseases. Do *NOT* mix up spine with spinal cord, especially in clinics or in the operating room.

A. Lumbar Strain

Buzz Words: Low back pain immediately after physical activity + no history of low blood pressure (LBP) proceeding + negative w/u

Clinical Presentation: The shelf exam will most likely test you on the management of a lumbar strain. Remember that the recommendation is to resume normal activity (and not to rest), because data show that the vast majority of low back pain is self-limiting and could be made worse/stiff with immobility.

PPx:
1. Avoid strenuous activity

MoD: Mechanical stress (lifting something too heavy)

Dx:
1. No need to image unless pain does not resolve
2. R/o radiculopathy with straight leg raise

Tx/Mgmt:
1. Nonsteroidal antiinflammatory drugs (NSAIDs)
2. Resume normal activity but no strenuous activity (resting w/o any activity does not improve LBP)

B. Spondylolysis

Buzz Words: Low back pain + exacerbated by activity (hyperextension) + Scottie dog sign

Clinical Presentation: Spondylolysis refers to phenomenon of fractures that appear in the interarticular portion of vertebral bone.

PPx:
1. avoid strenuous activity

MoD: Repeated microtrauma, degenerative → fx of pars interarticularis

Dx:
1. XR to view pars interarticularis, oblique view to see the "Scottie dog sign," or a dog with a collar around its neck (Fig. 8.1)

Tx/Mgmt:
1. Conservative → NSAIDs; avoid physical activity

C. Spondylolisthesis

Buzz Words: Low back pain + exacerbated by activity + vertebral body slipped forward on x-ray +/− presence of spondylolysis

Clinical Presentation: Spondylolisthesis is the displacement of a vertebral body relative to the vertebral body beneath it

PPx:
1. Avoid strenuous activity

MoD: Trauma, degenerative → slippage of superior vertebral body over inferior vertebral body

Dx:
1. XR

"Scottie dog"

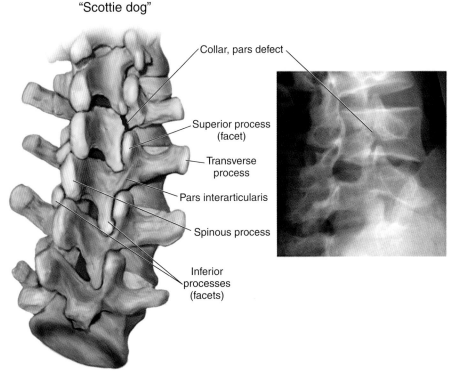

FIG. 8.1 Spondylolysis and "Scottie the dog." (From Miller M: *Miller's Review of orthopaedics*, ed 7. Philadelphia, 2016, Elsevier.)

Tx/Mgmt:
1. Conservative → NSAIDs, avoid physical activity
2. Cortisone
3. Spinal fusion

D. Spinal Stenosis

Buzz Words: Low back pain worse with activity + lower extremity pain + relieved by sitting and leaning forward (pushing a cart at the grocery store relieves back pain) + narrowing of canal on imaging + weakness/numbness of legs while walking → lumbar spinal stenosis

Neck pain/Upper back pain + radicular pain to arms + paresthesias/weakness of arm at compressed root → cervical spinal stenosis

• May get UMN signs of lower extremity if cervical stenosis is bad enough to cause myelopathy (spinal cord damage)

Weakness of upper extremity (UE; LMN at level of cervical spine) + hyper reflexivity/Babinski sign of lower extremities (UMN signs below level of cervical spine → Advanced cervical spinal stenosis)

Clinical Presentation: Spinal stenosis can be organized by the region of the spine. Cervical and lumbar regions are most common.

PPx: None

MoD: Congenital; degenerative, osteophytes in the vertebral canal → narrowing of canal

- Osteophytes are bony spurs that form next to each other 2/2 chronic degeneration.

Dx:
1. XR

Tx/Mgmt:
1. Conservative → NSAIDs, avoid physical activity
2. Cortisone

E. Cervical Disc Herniation

Buzz Words: Slipped disc C-spine + deltoid weakness + loss of shoulder sensation/upper lateral arm → C5 root impinged 2/2 C4-C5 disc herniation

Slipped disc C-spine + wrist extensor weakness + first/second finger numbness → C6 root impinged 2/2 C5-C6 disc herniation

Slipped disc c-spine + triceps weakness + triceps areflexia + middle finger numbness → C7 root impinged 2/2 C6-C7 disc herniation

Clinical Presentation: Cervical disc herniation is characterized by displacement of an intervertebral disc at the level of the C-spine, thereby impinging the nerve root one level inferior (e.g., slipped disc at C4-C5 would impinge C5).

PPx:
1. Avoid strenuous activity.

MoD: Degeneration of annulus fibrosis (usually posterolateral)

Dx:
1. XR

Tx/Mgmt:
1. Conservative → NSAIDs
2. Cortisone
3. Surgery

F. Lumbosacral Disc Herniation

Buzz Words: Slipped disc L-spine + iliopsoas/quad weakness + decreased patellar tendon reflex + numbness of knee → L4 root impingement 2/2 L3-L4 disc herniation

Slipped disc L-spine + weakness with foot dorsiflexion, eversion, inversion + numbness of dorsal foot → L5 root impingement 2/2 L4-L5 disc herniation

Slipped disc L-spine + weakness w/ foot planar flexion + loss of Achilles tendon reflex (ankle jerk) + loss of sensation of lateral foot/sole → S1 root impingement 2/2 L5-S1 disc herniation

Clinical Presentation: Characterized by displacement of an intervertebral disc at level of L-spine-spine; impinges nerve root at one level inferior (e.g., slipped disc at L3-L4 would impinge L4)

PPx:

1. Avoid strenuous activity.

MoD: Degeneration of annulus fibrosis (usually posterolateral) → intervertebral disc slippage

Dx:

1. Straight leg test (positive **only** if radicular pain; i.e., pain that shoots down leg)
2. XR

Tx/Mgmt:

1. Conservative → NSAIDs
2. Cortisone
3. Surgery

G. Ankylosing Spondylitis

Buzz Words: Morning stiffness + stiffness better w/ activity + bamboo spine on XR + pain at Achilles tendon (enthesitis) + sacroiliac joint stiffness

Clinical Presentation: Commonly tested because of its characteristic chief complaints (morning stiffness and bamboo spine on XR). Be prepared to identify bamboo spine on XR for the shelf.

PPx: None

MoD: Part of seronegative spondyloarthropathies (including Reiter syndrome aka reactive arthritis and psoriatic arthritis) → associated with HLA-B27

Dx:

1. XR
2. Rheumatoid factor to r/o RA

Tx/Mgmt:

1. NSAIDs
2. Physical therapy

H. Osteomyelitis of vertebra

Buzz Words: Back pain + tenderness to palpation at level of osteomyelitic bone + fever

Clinical Presentation: Osteomyelitis is an infection of the bone. Infectious agents, such as tuberculosis, can invade the vertebral body.

PPx: Avoid dirty needles

MoD: Hematogenous spread of bacteria to vertebral column
Dx:
1. XR
Tx/Mgmt:
1. Abx
2. Surgery

I. Compression Fracture of Vertebra
Buzz Words: LBP that is **well localized** + worse with activity
    + no fever
Clinical Presentation: Compression fracture has a similar
    presentation to osteomyelitis of spine but does not
    have fever or signs of systemic infection
PPx: None
MoD: Traumatic mechanism to spine
Dx:
1. XR
Tx/Mgmt:
1. Conservative → brace, NSAIDs, rest
2. Surgery

Disorders of the Spinal Cord

This section describes pathology pertaining to the spinal cord, which contains all of the nervous system communication between the brain and the PNS and its own intrinsic organization. The most commonly tested concept is cauda equina syndrome because of its emergent nature. Be able to differentiate cauda equina from conus medullaris by the end of this chapter. Also, be able to recognize the etiology of mixed UMN and LMN signs at different levels (spinal cord compression). Finally, know the term **autonomic dysreflexia**, which is a condition that is commonly seen in patients with a spinal cord injury at T6 or above, as the autonomic sympathetic system arises from this portion of spinal cord. Autonomic dysreflexia is 2/2 increased sympathetic discharge after an injury at or above T6, so patients would present with life-threatening hypertension and tachycardia.

99 AR

Autonomic Dysreflexia in Spinal
Cord Injury

A. Cauda Equina Syndrome
Buzz Words: Gradual low back pain that radiates down
    legs+ Asymmetric (worse on one side vs. the other) +
    decreased knee jerk + decreased ankle jerk + impotence + urinary retention
Clinical Presentation: Cauda equina syndrome is caused by
    compression of L2-S1 nerve roots, which leads to loss

of knee jerk reflex. Unlike conus medullaris, patients with cauda equina demonstrate **asymmetric** neurologic deficits.

MoD: Trauma, compression by mass (malignancy or abscess) → compression of cauda equina

Dx:

1. Emergent magnetic resonance imaging (MRI)

Tx/Mgmt:

1. Emergent condition → consult neurosurg asap (wake attending up)
2. Surgery to decompress cauda equine

Cauda Equina and Conus Medullaris Syndromes Clinical Presentation

B. Conus Medullaris Syndrome

Buzz Words: Sudden + symmetric (both legs) + decreased ankle jerk (S1) + knee jerk intact + impotence + urinary retention

Clinical Presentation: Conus medullaris is the end portion of the spinal cord and affects L5, S1-3. When there is no compression to the nerve roots of these levels, it may just lead to sensory loss in the genital region, loss of bladder control, and erectile function. If there is compression, may present as low back pain +/− weakness in the legs. Usually symmetric with no radicular pain. Knee jerk is intact because conus medullaris does not affect L3, L4

MoD: Trauma, compression by mass (malignancy or abscess) → compression of cauda equina

Dx:

1. Emergent MRI

Tx/Mgmt:

1. Emergent condition → consult neurosurg asap (wake attending up)
2. Surgery to decompress spinal cord

C. Anterior Spinal Artery (ASA) Syndrome

Buzz Words: Weakness + decreased pain and sensory loss (clear-cut sensory level of impairment, such as below T10 level) + preserved vibration/proprioception + in s/o surgery (particularly abdominal aortic aneurysmal repair)

Clinical Presentation: Very high-yield on the shelf. You will likely be asked what arterial branch was damaged during surgery that led to ASA syndrome (e.g., Adamkiewicz).

PPx:

1. Don't nick adjacent arteries during surgery.

MoD: Lesion of artery of **Adamkiewicz** during surgery, which is the largest branch of the ASA

Dx: None
Tx/Mgmt: None

D. Spinal Cord Compression (Myelopathy)

Buzz Words: LMN signs at level of compression + UMN signs below level of compression

Clinical Presentation: This topic is frequently tested on the neurology shelf because it can mimic amyotrophic lateral sclerosis (in both, patients can have both LMN and UMN signs). The biggest difference is that in spinal cord compression, the LMN and UMN signs are separated between upper and lower extremity. If the lesion is above the level of T6, be aware of **autonomic dysreflexia.** This can also occur in patients with rheumatoid etiology.

PPx: None

MoD: Due to anything that compresses the spinal cord, including spinal stenosis (mentioned previously) and masses

Dx:

1. Cervical XR

Tx/Mgmt: Depends on etiology; if degenerative → conservative Tx w/ pain meds first then surgery; if traumatic/infectious → steroids to reduce swelling, surgery

E. Anterior Cord Syndrome

Buzz Words: Loss of pain/temp bilaterally below lesion + LMN weakness below lesion + proprioception/vibration preserved +/− incontinence → anterior cord syndrome (Fig. 8.2)

Clinical Presentation: Anterior cord syndrome is the result of an occlusion of the ASA, whereas ASA syndrome is the result of an occlusion of a **branch** of the ASA.

PPx: None

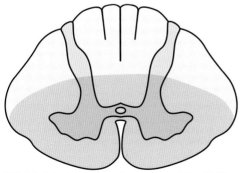

FIG. 8.2 Anterior cord syndrome. (From Winn H: *Youman's neurological surgery*, ed 6. Philadelphia, 2011, Elsevier.)

MoD: Due to anything that compresses the spinal cord anteriorly, including but not limited to trauma, abscess, malignancy, *or* due to lesion of the ASA (i.e., artery of Adamkiewicz during AAA surgery)

Dx:
1. XR
2. MRI if concerned for cauda equina

Tx/Mgmt: Depends on etiology; if traumatic/infectious → steroids to reduce swelling, surgery

F. Central Cord Syndrome

Buzz Words: Loss of pain/temp in "cape distribution" bilaterally over arms + no other lesions → small central cord syndrome (Fig. 8.3)

Loss of pain/temp, position/vibration + weakness below level of lesion → large central cord

Clinical Presentation: Most commonly presents as a middle-aged man or woman who loses pain and temperature sensation in a cape-like distribution over the upper extremities.

PPx: None

MoD: Can be caused by syringomyelia (most common), tumors, trauma. Most commonly syringomyelia → starting from center of spinal cord compresses spinothalamic tract crossing in the ventral commissure
• Expansion of syringomyelia starts to affect spinothalamic, corticospinal, and posterior column tracts.

Dx:
1. XR
2. MRI if concerned for cauda equina

Tx/Mgmt: Depends on etiology; if traumatic/infectious/neoplastic → steroids to reduce swelling, surgery

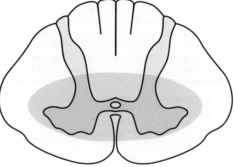

FIG. 8.3 Central cord syndrome. (From Winn H: *Youman's neurological surgery*, ed 6. Philadelphia, 2011, Elsevier.)

G. Posterior Cord syndrome

Buzz Words: Loss of position/vibration at or below level of lesion + no other focal abnormalities → posterior cord syndrome (Fig. 8.4)

Clinical Presentation: Can be differentiated from other spinal cord syndromes by the loss of functions carried out by the dorsal column

PPx: None

MoD: Can be caused by multiple sclerosis (MS), tumors, trauma, and vitamin B12 deficiency (subacute combined spinal cord syndrome — post cord and lateral cord)

Dx:

1. XR
2. MRI if concerned for MS

Tx/Mgmt: Treat depending on etiology (for instance, replenish with vitamin B12 if deficient).

H. Brown-Sequard Syndrome

Buzz Words: Ipsilateral loss of position/vibration + contralateral loss of pain/temp + contralateral weakness (Fig. 8.5)

Clinical Presentation: Brown-Sequard is defined as cord hemisection leading to sensory and motor dissociation.

PPx: None

MoD: Can be caused by MS, tumors, penetrating injuries (trauma is most common cause)

Dx:

1. XR
2. MRI if concerned for MS

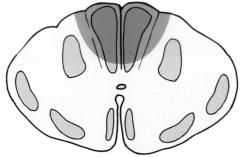

FIG. 8.4 Posterior cord syndrome. (Modified from Klein GR, Vaccaro AR: Cervical spine trauma: upper and lower. In Vaccaro AR, Betz RR, Zeidman SM, editors: *Principles and practice of spine surgery*, Philadelphia, 2003, Mosby, p 442. As adapted in Chen MN, Thorpe SW, Lee JY. Management of traumatic bilateral jumped cervical facet joints in a patient with incomplete myelopathy. In Benzel EC, editor: *Spine surgery*, ed 3, Philadelphia, 2012, Saunders, pp e2155–e2166.)

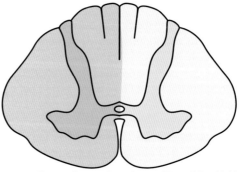

FIG. 8.5 Brown-Sequard syndrome. (From Winn H: *Youman's neurological surgery*, ed 6. Philadelphia, 2011, Elsevier.)

Tx/Mgmt:
1. Treat depending on etiology (for instance, prednisone for MS)

I. Malignant compression of spinal cord
Buzz Words: LBP + **pain at night** + weight loss + night sweats
Clinical Presentation: Patients with malignancy of the spine will often present with back pain accompanied by alarm signs/symptoms, such as pain that wakes them up at night as well as unexpected weight loss.
PPx: None
MoD: Tumors that metastasize to back, such as prostate cancer tumors
Dx:
1. XR
2. MRI and CT
Tx/Mgmt:
1. Prednisone to relieve swelling
2. Tx of primary cancer (surgery, chemo, radiation)

GUNNER PRACTICE

1. An 82-year-old woman comes to the physician because of a 1-year history of neck stiffness, pain radiating from her neck to her left hand, urinary incontinence, and unsteadiness with walking. Past medical history includes osteoarthritis, peptic ulcer disease, and hyperlipidemia. Current medications are naproxen, ranitidine, and lovastatin. She has a history of alcohol abuse but has abstained from drinking for 5 years. Neurologic examination shows atrophy of the left upper extremity and increased tone in both lower extremities. Muscle

strength in the left upper extremity is 3/5. Deep tendon reflexes are 2+ at the biceps and brachioradialis bilaterally, absent at the left triceps and 3+ at the knees and ankles. Babinski sign is present bilaterally. Sensitivity to pinprick and temperature is decreased over the left dorsal forearm and hand. Proprioception and sensitivity to vibration are markedly decreased at the ankles and toes. She has a stiff wide-based gait. Which of the following is the most likely diagnosis?

A. Bilateral brachial plexopathy
B. Epidural cord compression
C. Parasagittal meningioma
D. Peripheral neuropathy
E. Spondylotic cervical myelopathy

ANSWERS: What Would Gunner Jess/Jim Do?

1. WWGJD? An 82-year-old woman comes to the physician because of a 1-year history of neck stiffness, pain radiating from her neck to her left hand, urinary incontinence, and unsteadiness with walking. Past medical history includes osteoarthritis, peptic ulcer disease, and hyperlipidemia. Current medications are naproxen, ranitidine, and lovastatin. She has a history of alcohol abuse but has abstained from drinking for 5 years. Neurologic examination shows atrophy of the left upper extremity and increased tone in both lower extremities. Muscle strength in the left upper extremity is 3/5. Deep tendon reflexes are 2+ at the biceps and brachioradialis bilaterally, absent at the left triceps and 3+ at the knees and ankles. Babinski sign is present bilaterally. Sensation to pinprick and temperature is decreased over left dorsal forearm and hand. Proprioception and sensation to vibration are markedly decreased at the ankles and toes. She has a stiff wide-based gait. Which of the following is the most likely diagnosis?

Answer: E, Spondylotic cervical myelopathy

Explanation: This is a classic example of cervical spondylotic myelopathy (aka disease of the spinal cord). Spondylotic cervical myelopathy is a neck condition in which the cervical spinal cord is compressed due to degenerative changes in the vertebral column (e.g., osteophytes in the vertebral column). Compression of the spinal cord will result in LMN signs (areflexia and weakness/numbness) at the level of compression, as well as UMN signs below the level of compression. This can be seen in the question stem. The patient has areflexia of the "left triceps" and weakness in left upper extremity ("3/5" in muscle strength), which are LMN signs of C7 compression on the left side. The patient also has "Babinski sign...present bilaterally" and "increased tone" in both lower extremities, both of which are UMN signs. Therefore the choices should be narrowed to E and B, epidural cord compression.

To differentiate cervical myelopathy from epidural cord compression, look at the timeline. The patient has had "neck stiffness" for "1 year" and does not have exam signs suggesting malignancy (e.g., weight loss) or infection (e.g., fever). Thus epidural cord compression is less likely and E can be selected as the answer.

   A. Bilateral brachial plexopathy → Incorrect. All of the upper extremity symptoms affected the left side. Thus it doesn't make sense for "bilateral" brachial plexuses to be involved. Also, brachial plexopathy would not lead to lower extremity signs and symptoms.

B. Epidural cord compression → Incorrect. This answer choice would be correct if the timeline were more acute (e.g., <1 month) and the patient had signs of something compressing the spinal cord (e.g., malignancy as evidenced by weight loss/pain that wakes the patient up at night, or abscess as evidenced by fever/tenderness to palpation).

C. Parasagittal meningioma → Incorrect. Meningioma located parasagittally in the cerebrum would not lead to LMN signs (i.e., the areflexia seen in the left biceps). It would only lead to UMN signs.

D. Peripheral neuropathy → Incorrect. The fact that the patient has a positive "Babinski sign" should automatically lead you to think *UMN lesion.* By definition, UMNs reside in the CNS and do not fall under the domain of "peripheral neuropathy."

9

Traumatic, Mechanical, and Intracranial Pressure Disorders in the Neurology Shelf

Hao-Hua Wu, Leo Wang, and Chuang-Kuo Wu

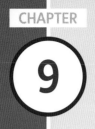

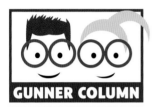

GUNNER COLUMN

This chapter is divided into two parts. In the first section, you will learn about head and neck trauma. This is an important section because many of these disorders, such as epidural hematoma and uncal herniation, are emergent and thus frequently tested across all shelf exams (i.e. neuro, medicine, surgery, etc.) and Step 2 CK. Thus if this is your first shelf exam, it would behoove you to learn this section well. If you have already seen this material on another rotation, it won't hurt to get a little bit of a refresher. Of note, most of the disorders in this section lead to an **acute** rise in intracranial pressure (ICP). One of the organizing themes to learn is how to treat an acute rise in ICP.

The second section is dedicated to disorders that lead to a **chronic** rise in ICP. These disorders include the frequently tested idiopathic intracranial hypertension (IIH; aka pseudotumor cerebri) and normal pressure hydrocephalus. These disorders also come up again and again on multiple shelf exams, so learn them well. Focus particularly on the buzz words that will allow you to reach a quick diagnosis after reading a long NBME question stem.

Head and Neck Trauma

One of the key principles is knowing how to decrease ICP and how quickly each step decreases ICP, as the shelf often asks which method is the quickest way to decrease ICP. These are the steps to decrease ICP in order of quickest to longest:

Step	Time to Decrease ICP
Reverse Trendelenburg position of bed (elevate head of bed above 45 degrees)	Immediate
Hyperventilation and intubation	30 s

Step	Time to Decrease ICP
IV Mannitol or hypertonic saline → Na >138 or osmolarity 300–310 w/normal BP	5 min (furosemide can also be added)
Ventricular drainage	Minutes
Barbiturate induced coma	1 h (2/2 vasoconstriction of cerebrum and reduced metabolic demands)
Steroids	Hours

The only exception to the list is if the increase in ICP is 2/2 a mass (abscess or malignancy), then jump to #6 on this list with dexamethasone to reduce inflammation. Focal or hemicraniotomy can also be used to immediately reduce ICP, but that is only done in case of emergency (like epidural hematoma). Otherwise, memorize this order, and you are guaranteed to answer one or two shelf exam questions correctly (as this also shows up on the surgery shelf).

Another organizing principle is to recognize the signs and symptoms of increased ICP. First, the body will respond by pupillary dilation on the side of hemorrhage and papilledema. The body then responds to the increased ICP with the Cushing reflex → include hypertension + bradycardia + irregular respiration.

Be wary of patients with photophobia, stiff neck, and dilated pupils. The former two symptoms are associated with meningitis, but the presence of dilated pupils means that it is in fact a hemorrhage/aneurysmal rupture rather than meningitis driving the disease process. Subarachnoid hemorrhage can present like meningitis minus the fever!

Lastly, herniation disorders are included here because they are often the sequelae of untreated head trauma 2/2 hemorrhage mass effect.

A. Epidural Hematoma

Buzz Words: Fixed dilated pupil (if already causing ipsilateral uncal herniation) + contralateral hemiparesis + biconvex/lens-shaped hematoma + lucid interval (Fig. 9.1)

Clinical Presentation: Epidural hematoma is high-yield on the shelf and is characterized by a lucid interval (when the patient's mental state improves shortly after trauma, only to worsen later on). Make sure to know what an epidural hematoma looks like on noncontrast head computed tomography (CT) scans. Patients with head

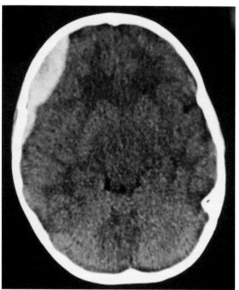

FIG. 9.1 Head computed tomography of epidural hematoma. (From Huisman TAGM, Tschirch FTC: Epidural hematoma in children: do cranial structures act as a barrier? *J Neuroradiol.* 36(2):93–97, 2008.)

trauma frequently get head CT's first to rule out epidural/subdural hematomas.

PPx: None

MoD: Traumatic injury (bike accident without a helmet, etc.) → fracture of temporal bone → rupture of the middle meningeal artery in the epidural space

Dx:

1. CT/magnetic resonance imaging (MRI) will show crescent-shaped hematoma; the bleeding region is limited by the skull suture line (the most important radiographic finding)
2. X-ray of cervical spine to r/o injury

Tx/Mgmt:

1. Emergent craniotomy
2. Ventriculostomy for ICP monitoring

B. Subdural Hematoma

Buzz Words:

- Large trauma + does not have to be old + obtunded/no lucid interval + semilunar/crescent-shaped hematoma → acute subdural hematoma (Fig. 9.2)
- Very old + alcoholics + shrunken brain rattled by minor trauma + altered mental status → chronic subdural hematoma

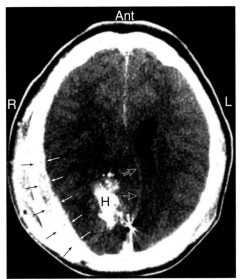

FIG. 9.2 Head computed tomography of subdural hematoma. (From Mettler FA, editor: *Primary care radiology*, Philadelphia, 2000, Saunders.)

Clinical Presentation: Subdural hematomas are also high-yield. Oftentimes you will be expected to make the diagnosis based on an axial noncontrast head CT. As opposed to epidural hematoma, subdural hematomas have a semilunar shape.

PPx: None

MoD: Traumatic injury → tearing of **bridging veins** as they cross from subdural space into dura

Dx:
1. CT/MRI will show crescent shaped hematoma (crossing the surface of brain)
2. XR of cervical spine to r/o injury

Tx/Mgmt:
1. If midline deviated → craniotomy or ventriculostomy
2. If not deviated → decrease ICP (i.e., elevate head, hyperventilate, avoid fluid overload, mannitol)
3. Hypothermia to reduce oxygen demand of brain

C. Basal Skull Fracture

Buzz Words: Raccoon eyes + rhinorrhea + otorrhea + ecchymosis behind the ear (Battle sign)

Clinical Presentation: Basal skull fractures are commonly tested on the neurology and surgery shelf. You may be shown a picture of a patient with either a Battle sign or "raccoon eyes."

PPx: None

MoD: Traumatic injury

Dx:

1. Physical exam (look for Battle sign)
2. CT head/neck
3. Cervical XR to r/o spinal injury

Tx/Mgmt:

1. Neurosurgery consultation for possible surgical intervention

D. Traumatic Brain Injury (TBI)

Buzz Words:

- Diffuse blurring of gray-white matter interface + multiple small punctate hemorrhages + severe trauma → **severe** traumatic brain injury 2/2 diffuse axonal injury (contusion and DAI)
- Loss of consciousness + confusion + <2 hours + normal MRI/CT + difficulty with memory (anterograde, retrograde) + headache → mild TBI
- Headaches + lethargy + mental dullness + months after initial trauma → concussion and postconcussive syndrome

Clinical Presentation: Traumatic brain injury refers to the spectrum of injury caused to the brain by traumatic force. A mild traumatic brain injury is a "concussion." A moderate to severe traumatic brain injury is a "contusion."

PPx: None

MoD: Comes from stretching of the axons 2/2 traumatic force

Dx:

1. CT/MRI to r/o hematoma
2. XR of cervical spine to r/o spinal injury

Tx/Mgmt:

1. Prevention of ICP increase
2. Surgery if accompanying expanding hematoma that worsens ICP
   - Supportive care; no direct treatment protocol right now that directly address TBI

E. Dementia Pugilistica

Buzz Words: Pro boxers and NFL players—History of concussions, head injury + memory loss + no other family history of Alzheimer's, Parkinson's

Clinical Presentation: Dementia pugilistica is characterized by memory loss from repeated concussions with/without contusion

PPx: Avoid head trauma

MoD: Unknown

Dx:
1. UDS to r/o medication/drug induced dementia
2. CT/MRI to r/o vascular dementia

Tx/Mgmt: None

F. Transtentorial (aka Uncal) Herniation

Buzz Words: Head trauma + blown pupil + down and out eye + hemiparesis (ipsilateral or contralateral) + coma

Clinical Presentation: Uncal herniation is defined by a triad of hemiplegia, coma, and blown pupil (from cranial nerve [CN] III palsy). Herniation occurs when there is enough **mass effect** to push intracranial structures from one place to another. Mass effect is the term to describe a phenomenon when a large lesion (i.e., tumor, hemorrhage, abscess) develops pressure to shift intracranial structures.

PPx: None

MoD: Mass effect → herniation of the medial temporal lobe, especially the uncus of the medial temporal lobe → compresses CN III nerve (blown pupil), cerebral peduncle (contralateral hemiparesis) or corticospinal tract of midbrain (ipsilateral hemiparesis; aka Kernohan phenomenon) and reticular activating formation of midbrain (coma)

Dx:
1. CT scan

Tx/Mgmt:
1. Decompressive craniectomy

G. Central Herniation

Buzz Words: Head trauma + CN VI palsy + elevated ICP

Clinical Presentation: Central herniation is herniation of the brainstem downward (a cone force from superior tentorium to inferior tentorium). It can also lead to symptoms of uncal herniation if the central herniation is big enough.

PPx: None

MoD: Increased ICP (e.g., pseudotumor cerebri) → central herniation

Dx:
1. CT scan/brain MRI can detect this condition better with a sagittal view

Tx/Mgmt:
1. Decompressive craniectomy

H. Tonsillar Herniation

Buzz Words: Head trauma + respiratory arrest + blood pressure (BP) instability + death

Clinical Presentation: Tonsillar herniation occurs when there is a herniation of cerebellar tonsils downward through the foramen magnum, leading to pressure placed on the lower brainstem (medullary portion).

PPx: None

MoD: Can be precipitated by low pressure (LP) in a patient with significantly elevated ICP above the level of the cerebellar tonsils

- That's why a CT is done before an LP

Dx: CT scan/brain MRI can detect this condition clearly

Tx/Mgmt: Decompressive craniectomy

I. Subfalcine Herniation

Buzz Words: Head trauma + Infarct of the ACA (lower extremity weakness/sensory loss, frontal lobe behaviors) + herniation on CT

Clinical Presentation: Subfalcine herniation occurs when there is herniation of brain structures (e.g., cingulate gyrus) under the falx cerebri.

PPx: None

MoD: Mass effect → subfalcine herniation

Dx:

1. CT scan
2. MRI for ACA vessels

Tx/Mgmt:

1. Decompressive craniectomy

J. Torticollis

Buzz Words: Fixed rotation of neck to one side + pediatric patient

Clinical Presentation: Torticollis can be seen as a result of trauma from delivery, a retropharyngeal abscess, or an upper respiratory infection. It is considered a mechanical disorder on the neurology shelf based on the NBME organization, although it is classically grouped with movement disorders.

PPx: None

MoD: Could be 2/2 URI *OR* minor trauma *OR* cervical lymphadenitis *OR* retropharyngeal abscess

Dx:

1. Cervical spine radiographs (XR of neck) to r/o cervical spine fracture or dislocation
2. Retropharyngeal abscess
3. Atlantoaxial subluxation

Tx/Mgmt:

1. With soft neck collar (for MSK torticollis)

K. Cervical Dystonia (aka Spasmodic Torticollis)

Buzz Words: Adult patient + neck keeps turning to one side episodically+ chronic timeline (>3 months) + cervical muscles tense on exam + rest of exam normal

Clinical Presentation: Cervical dystonia is differentiated from torticollis by patient age. Like torticollis, cervical dystonia is frequently taught in the category of "movement disorder," although the NBME classifies this entity as a mechanical disorder.

PPx: None

MoD: Idiopathic (likely neurological)

Dx:
1. Physical exam
2. Cervical spine radiographs (XR of neck) to r/o cervical spine fracture or dislocation

Tx/Mgmt:
1. Analgesics for pain
2. **Botulinum toxin** to relax muscles

Disorders of Increased Intracranial Pressure (ICP)

These disorders are more subacute or chronic disorders (>1 month in course/duration). Thus measures like Trendelenburg or hyperventilation aren't as important for the patient, since disease processes like pseudotumor cerebri are not immediately life threatening. Instead, treatment measures for these disorders of increased ICP require longer term therapy.

The reason why it is so important to decrease ICP is that increased ICP means less cerebral blood flow. There is an equation that states the cerebral perfusion pressure (CPP) is equal to the mean arterial pressure minus the ICP—that is, $CPP = MAP - ICP$. Thus as ICP increases and CPP stays the same, the MAP would have to decrease. A decreased MAP in the setting of increased ICP means less cerebral blood flow.

This section also covers hydrocephalus. Hydrocephalus means excess CSF in the intracranial cavity. This can be caused by (1) excess CSF production, (2) obstruction of flow at any point in ventricles or subarachnoid space, and (3) decreased reabsorption through arachnoid granulations. It would be good to know the hydrocephalus disorders that are caused by excess production (e.g., tumors such as choroid plexus papilloma) and obstruction (e.g., intracranial hemorrhage, congenital malformations). Since decreased CSF reabsorption is difficult to ascertain clinically, hydrocephalus disorders are broken down into (1) communicating hydrocephalus (aka nonobstructive hydrocephalus) and (2) noncommunicating hydrocephalus (aka obstructive hydrocephalus → obstruction of CSF flow in the ventricular system).

A. Idiopathic Intracranial Hypertension (IIH; aka Pseudotumor Cerebri)

Buzz Words:
- Young woman + headache + papilledema on exam + hx of vitamin A intake + slit-like ventricles on CT → idiopathic intracranial hypertension
- Young woman + headache + sixth nerve palsies + tinnitus + visual disturbances + papilledema → IIH
- Untreated IIH → blindness

Clinical Presentation: Pseudotumor cerebri is a high-yield topic on the shelf. In particular, it is associated with a history of vitamin A intake and should be first on the differential for any female patient who presents with a headache and papilledema.

PPx: (1) Avoid oral contraceptives and vitamin A intake.

MoD: Idiopathic (hence the name)

Dx:
1. Fundoscopic exam to look for papilledema
2. MRI/CT to r/o mass (must do before lumbar puncture to avoid herniation)
3. Spinal tap (aka lumbar puncture) will show elevated CSF pressure but normal CSF analysis.

Tx/Mgmt:
1. Acetazolamide to reduce CSF
2. Furosemide
3. Spinal tap (repeated over time)
4. Optic nerve fenestration to reduce risk of damage to optic nerve
5. Ventriculo-peritoneal shunting (V-P) or spinal-peritoneal shunting

B. Normal Pressure Hydrocephalus (NPH)

Buzz Words: Has difficulty walking + urinary incontinence + mental decline

Clinical Presentation: The NPH triad is wet (urinary incontinence), wobbly (cannot walk; so-called magnetic gait or gait apraxia), and weird (memory loss). Since this is such a frequently tested topic for the neuro shelf, the test writers get **very creative** when it comes to describing these three symptoms. For instance, a patient's

QUICK TIPS

Wet, wobbly, and weird = NPH

relative could describe the patient as "hasn't been able to hold it in recently," and one would have to ascertain the "wet" symptom of the triad.

PPx: None

MoD: Defective superior sagittal sinus → clogged arachnoid granulations → communicating hydrocephalus → stretching of the corona radiata

Dx:
1. CT
2. LP (likely show normal pressure CSF)

Tx/Mgmt:
1. Serial LPs
2. Ventriculoperitoneal shunting

C. Obstructive Hydrocephalus

Buzz Words: mass effect + headache + N/V + cognitive impairment + papilledema + CN VI palsy → potential obstructive hydrocephalus

Clinical Presentation: Obstructive hydrocephalus is not a specific disorder, but rather a unifying outcome caused by many different disease processes (e.g., hemorrhage, tumor, etc.).

PPx: None

MoD: Can be due to tumors, hemorrhage, congenital malformations that block the ventricular system, particularly at the levels of foramen of Monro of the lateral ventricle, midbrain aqueduct, and opening of fourth ventricle

Dx:
1. CT

Tx/Mgmt:
1. External ventricular drain
2. Ventriculoperitoneal shunt
3. Endoscopic neurosurgery

D. Parinaud Syndrome

Buzz Words: Inability to gaze upward + bilateral deviation of the eyes downward and inward + headache

Clinical Presentation: Parinaud syndrome is a very unique disorder tested on the shelf, as it involves the pineal recess. Patients present with an inability to gaze upward. It is likely a sequela of enlarging hydrocephalus.

PPx: None

MoD: Dilation of the supra-pineal recess of posterior third ventricle → push downward onto the collicular plate of the midbrain → Parinaud syndrome

Dx: CT/MRI

Tx/Mgmt:
1. External ventricular drain
2. Ventriculoperitoneal shunt
3. Endoscopic neurosurgery

E. Hydrocephalus ex Vacuo

Buzz Words: N/A

Clinical Presentation: Not actually a disease process. Describes the appearance of enlarged ventricles or dilated ventricles that are most commonly due to brain tissue atrophy. Can be seen in degenerative disorders like Alzheimer's. This term was put in the hydrocephalus region to dispel the confusion and clarify that although there is "hydrocephalus" in the name, "hydrocephalus ex vacuo" is not true hydrocephalus.

PPx: N/A

MoD: N/A

Dx: N/A

Tx/Mgmt: N/A

GUNNER PRACTICE

1. A 61-year-old man is brought immediately to the hospital after his wife finds him unconscious. Past medical history is significant for hypertension. He withdraws the left extremities vigorously to painful stimuli, but there is no movement of the right arm or leg. He moans incomprehensibly and opens his eyes briefly to noxious stimuli. His temperature is 37°C (98.6°F), pulse is 60/min, respirations are 10/min, and BP is 192/86. The left pupil is 6 mm and nonreactive, and the right pupil is 3 mm and reactive to light. Fundoscopic examination shows no abnormalities. Deep tendon reflexes are absent in the right extremities, and Babinski sign is also present on the right. Which of the following will most rapidly decrease the patient's intracranial pressure?
   A. Trendelenburg (head down) positioning
   B. IV dexamethasone therapy
   C. IV mannitol therapy
   D. Oral glycerol therapy through nasogastric tube
   E. Intubation and hyperventilation

2. After nearly drowning after a major accident in a swimming pool, a 65-year-old woman develops severe hypoxia with accompanying edema in her brain, which elevates her intracranial pressure. On imaging, you find that the medial temporal lobe has begun to compress

on the tentorium cerebelli. Which clinical finding would be associated with this imaging result?

A. Both pupils 5–6 mm and fixed
B. Anisocoria ipsilateral to compression
C. External oculomotor ophthalmoplegia
D. Anisocoria contralateral to compression
E. Ptosis contralateral to compression

3. A 65-year-old woman is brought to the physician by her husband because of a 6-month history of memory problems and urinary incontinence. He says that she continues to forget to turn off the stove when cooking, and once forgot to turn off the bathtub water. Physical exam shows nystagmus, and you notice broad-based gait when she walks into the room. Neurologic exam shows no abnormalities. Her mini-mental status exam score is 18/30. Which of the following is the most appropriate next step in diagnosis?

A. CT scan
B. Head MRI
C. Lumbar puncture
D. Thoracic spine x-rays
E. Cervical spine x-rays

ANSWERS: What Would Gunner Jess/Jim Do?

1. WWGJD? A 61-year-old man is brought immediately to the hospital after his wife found him unconscious. Past medical history is significant for hypertension. He withdraws the left extremities vigorously to painful stimuli, but there is no movement of the right arm or leg. He moans incomprehensibly and opens his eyes briefly to noxious stimuli. His temperature is 37C (98.6F), pulse is 60/min, respirations are 10/min, and BP is 192/86. The left pupil is 6mm and nonreactive, and the right pupil is 3 mm and reactive to light. Fundoscopic examination shows no abnormalities. Deep tendon reflexes are absent in the right extremities and Babinski sign is also present on the right. Which of the following will most rapidly decrease the patient's intracranial pressure?

Answer: E, Intubation and hyperventilation

Explanation: This is the answer because intubation/hyperventilation reduces ICP in 30 seconds, which is faster than the other answer choices. In fact, the only two things that are faster are the reverse Trendelenburg position (elevated head) and emergent craniectomy, which can both decrease ICP immediately. This question requires you to have the speed of ICP interventions memorized. Of note, a gunner way to look at this question is to just read the last sentence. Since the question asks for the fastest way to decrease intracranial pressure, you can ascertain the answer just by recalling the timing of interventions to decrease ICP, thus saving yourself an extra 30 seconds or so. For those of you who did read through the whole question stem, what is your diagnosis? If you answered uncal herniation, you are correct. This patient has the uncal herniation triad of coma ("unconscious in a pool of vomit"), blown pupil ("left pupil is 6 mm and nonreactive"), and hemiparesis ("no movement of the right arm or leg"). It is key to note how the question stem gives you these signs/symptoms without outright saying the words coma, blown pupil, or hemiparesis.

A. Trendelenburg (head down) positioning → Incorrect. May have been tempting to folks who read the answer choice too quickly. But remember, Trendelenburg means head **down**, which would actually **elevate** ICP (counterproductive). Instead, when there is increased ICP, the treatment is to decrease it by elevating the head and decreasing the ICP.

B. IV dexamethasone therapy → Incorrect. Also used to decrease ICP, especially in a patient with an inflammatory mass effect (e.g., tumor, infection). Since there is no mention of neuroimaging in this question stem, it is safe to assume that the herniation is 2/2 hemorrhage.

C. IV mannitol therapy → Incorrect. This is the step after hyperventilation and intubation. This would decrease ICP in 5 minutes

D. Oral glycerol therapy through nasogastric tube → Incorrect. Similar to mannitol in treatment, but rarely used. Thus the timing to decrease ICP is similar to mannitol but slower than intubation and hyperventilation.

2. **WWGJD?** After nearly drowning after a major accident in a swimming pool, a 65-year-old woman develops severe hypoxia with accompanying edema in her brain, which elevates her intracranial pressure. On imaging, you find that the medial temporal lobe has begun to compress on the tentorium cerebelli. Which clinical finding would be associated with this imaging result?

Answer: B, Anisocoria ipsilateral to compression

Explanation: Compression of the medial temporal lobe against the tentorium cerebelli leads to compression of cranial nerve III, which will lead to a fixed/dilated pupil ipsilateral to the site of compression due to an inability to constrict in response to light. Anisocoria is by definition unequal pupil sizes.

A. Both pupils 5–6 mm and fixed → Incorrect. Compression of CNIII (oculomotor) would not affect the contralateral pupil, and thus both pupils would not be equal in size nor fixed.

C. External oculomotor ophthalmoplegia → Incorrect. External oculomotor ophthalmoplegia would lead to double vision, diplopia, and an inability for the patient to move the eye normally commensurate with weakness in the extraocular muscles innervated by the oculomotor nerve.

D. Anisocoria contralateral to compression → Incorrect. The unaffected eye would be able to constrict in response to light and is therefore not anisocoric.

E. Ptosis contralateral to compression → Incorrect. Ptosis is caused by Horner syndrome or oculomotor nerve palsy, or can be myogenic (i.e., myasthenia gravis). Ptosis, if applicable, would appear ipsilateral to the lesion.

3. WWGJD? A 65-year-old woman is brought to the physician by her husband because of a 6-month history of memory problems and urinary incontinence. He says that she continues to forget to turn off the stove when cooking, and once forgot to turn off the bathtub water. Physical exam shows nystagmus, and you notice broad-based gait when she walks into the room. Neurologic exam shows no abnormalities. Her mini-mental status exam score is 18/30. Which of the following is the most appropriate next step in diagnosis?

Answer: A, CT scan

Explanation: This patient meets the typical presentation for normal pressure hydrocephalus, as indicated by the "wet, wobbly, and weird" signs that she exhibits (urinary incontinence, memory loss and forgetfulness, and gait ataxia). NPH is diagnosed with CT, which will display enlarged ventricles and sometimes cortical atrophy. This is followed by LP to show that opening pressure is normal.

B. Head MRI → Incorrect. MRI is not indicated, since ventricles can easily be visualized by CT.

C. Lumbar puncture → Incorrect. LP would be indicated only after the CT scan is already made. An LP without a CT (and with a regular opening pressure) serves no diagnostic value.

D. Thoracic spine X-rays → Incorrect. There is nothing to suggest any thoracic spine abnormalities.

E. Cervical spine X-rays → Incorrect. There is nothing to suggest any cervical spine abnormalities.

Disorders of the Cranial Nerves and Peripheral Nervous System

10

George Hung, Hao-Hua Wu, Leo Wang, and Chuang-Kuo Wu

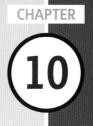

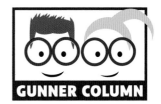

GUNNER COLUMN

This chapter covers the majority of disease processes one can expect to see pertaining to the peripheral nervous system (PNS), which along with the central nervous system (CNS), make up the nervous system as a whole. This section also covers Musculoskeletal System topics, which comprises a significant number of questions on the test.

In this chapter, peripheral nerve disorders are split into three sections: (1) cranial nerve injury/disorders, (2) peripheral nerve injury/disorders with an emphasis on plexus injuries, and (3) neurologic pain syndromes. Although neuromuscular disorders and movement disorders can also be lumped under peripheral nerve disorders, they are omitted from this chapter and will be presented individually in Chapters 16 and 17.

The emphasis in this chapter is on recognition of Buzz Words. For commonly tested disorders, such as Bell palsy, carpal tunnel syndrome (CTS), and Guillain-Barre syndrome (GBS), know the steps for diagnosis and treatment/management.

Perhaps the most important organizing principle is that symptoms derived from peripheral nerve disorders are of the lower motor neuron variety (i.e., fasciculations, weakness, areflexia, etc.). If you see any upper motor neuron (UMN) signs, such as Babinski sign or hyperreflexia, it means the CNS is involved.

While perusing this chapter, do not get frustrated if you have forgotten the anatomy or if you do not remember which nerve innervates what. Instead, use this as an opportunity to refer back to the "General Principles" chapter to refresh your understanding of anatomical concepts. The shelf exam is all about making connections to seemingly disparate areas of study. One way to keep yourself on track is to list the page numbers of pertinent anatomy next to the disease of interest. That way, you can easily refer to the correct page when lost.

This is a long chapter, so budget at least 5 hours for study.

Cranial Nerve Injury and Disorders

Cranial nerve injury was already covered to a large extent in Chapter 5, so if you are looking for vascular disorders of

the cranial nerves, refer to Chapter 5. This chapter, instead, deals with intrinsic injuries to the cranial nerves with etiologies ranging from idiopathic to infectious to traumatic.

A. Bell Palsy

Buzz Words:

- Hemiparesis of upper and lower face + can't make tears + hyperacusis + acute onset → Bell palsy
- Hemiparesis of upper and lower face + can't make tears + normal sensation + hyperacusis + gradual onset → Facial nerve tumor
- Bilateral Bell palsy + target rash + carditis (AV block, cardiomyopathy) + meningitis + migratory arthralgia + conjunctivitis + generalized LAD → Early disseminated Lyme disease (Lyme disease Bell palsy is usually bilateral)

Clinical Presentation: Bell Palsy is frequently tested and is characterized by unilateral paralysis of the face. Make sure to learn the Buzz Words of different disease processes that can lead to Bell palsy or Bell palsy-like presentation. The classic definition of Bell palsy is idiopathic, unilateral dysfunction of the motor branch of CN V2.

PPx: None

MoD: Bell palsy is an old term that was by definition idiopathic. Now it is one of a constellation of syndromes that lead to facial nerve palsy. Thus, questions that describe facial nerve lesions can be describing idiopathic Bell or palsy 2/2 herpes simplex, herpes zoster, facial nerve tumor, Lyme disease, or sarcoidosis.

- Also potentially caused by viral infections, including Coxsackie, CMV, adeno, etc.

Dx:

1. Lyme titer
2. CXR and serum ACE levels to rule out (r/o) sarcoidosis
3. Head computed tomography (CT)/brain magnetic resonance imaging (MRI) to r/o cerebellar-pontine (C-P) tumor
   - Bell palsy usually resolves on its own; if it doesn't, then proceed with steps 2 and 3

Tx/Mgmt:

1. Eye drops to avoid corneal abrasion
2. Steroids to reduce inflammation
3. Acyclovir if 2/2 herpes

B. Internuclear Ophthalmoplegia (INO)

Buzz Words:

- Loss of eye adduction on ipsilateral lateral gaze + nystagmus of the unaffected eye (CN6 overfires to stimulate CN3) + in s/o multiple sclerosis (MS), stroke → internuclearophthalmoplegia (INO)

- Eyes can still turn inward when focusing on a nearby object, but not when gazing laterally
- Ipsilateral eye motionless on lateral gaze + contralateral eye unable to gaze laterally + in s/o MS, stroke → One-and-a-half syndrome
- Eyes can still turn inward when focusing on a nearby object, but not when gazing laterally

Clinical Presentation: MoD of INO and one-and-a-half syndrome is the most frequently tested component on the shelf.

PPx: None

MoD: Lesion of the medial longitudinal fasciculus 2/2 stroke, multiple sclerosis, tumor, trauma, etc.

- Located medially next to cerebral aqueduct of the brainstem structures

In one-and-a-half syndrome, lesion is to the paramedian pontine reticular formation (PPRF) or VI nerve nucleus and MLF fibers crossing from contralateral VI nucleus.

Dx:
1. Extraocular movement eye exam
2. MRI to r/o MS and stroke

Tx/Mgmt:
1. Treat underlying condition (i.e., stroke Tx, MS Tx)
2. Patch one eye for symptomatic relief of diplopia

C. Vestibular Neuritis

Buzz Words: Sudden incapacitating vertigo + no hearing loss or tinnitus + less than 1-week duration

Clinical Presentation: Unlike labyrinthitis and Meniere disease, vestibular neuritis **does not** present with hearing loss and tinnitus.

PPx: None

MoD: Thought to be acute viral or postviral inflammatory disorder of vestibular portion of CN8

Dx:
1. History and physical (H&P)
2. Gadolinium-enhanced MRI

Tx/Mgmt:
1. Symptomatic/supportive treatments (e.g., antiemetics, fluids) since disease is self-resolving
2. Corticosteroids to speed recovery

D. Labyrinthitis

Buzz Words: Hearing loss + tinnitus + incapacitating vertigo + ear pain + fever

gg AR
MLF syndrome—Internuclear Ophthalmoplegia, Made Easy

gg AR
One-and-a-Half syndrome

gg AR
MLF Tutorial

Clinical Presentation: Labyrinthitis presents as sudden incapacitating vertigo as the predominant symptom, with variable degrees of hearing loss and tinnitus. Meniere presents as episodic vertigo, progressive or fluctuating sensorineural hearing loss, and tinnitus.

PPx: None

MoD: Thought to be bacterial or viral in origin, resulting in inflammation of vestibular and cochlear portions of CN8

Dx:

1. If unilateral hearing loss/tinnitus, gadolinium-enhanced MRI
2. If purulent infection suspected, temporal bone CT to r/o osteomyelitis and spread of infection

Tx/Mgmt:

1. Symptomatic/supportive measures (e.g., fluids, antipyretics)
2. Antibiotics

E. Horner Syndrome

Buzz Words:

- Drooping eyelid + no sweat + small pupil (<3 mm) → Horner syndrome (Fig. 10.1)
- Drooping eyelid + small pupil (<3 mm) + sweating of lower face normal → Horner syndrome 2/2 lesion of internal carotid (since sympathetic nerves to lower

99 AR
Horner Syndrome

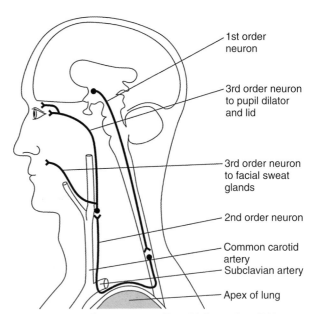

1st order neuron

3rd order neuron to pupil dilator and lid

3rd order neuron to facial sweat glands

2nd order neuron

Common carotid artery

Subclavian artery

Apex of lung

FIG. 10.1 Horner syndrome anatomy. (From McGee, editor: *Evidence-based physical diagnosis*. ed 3. Philadelphia, 2012, Saunders.)

face sweat glands out at external carotid at 3rd-order neuron)

Clinical Presentation: The Buzz Words of Horner syndrome are easily recognized. Thus to trick you, the shelf will test on the mechanism (i.e., lesion at 1st-order vs. 2nd-order vs. 3rd-order neuron).

PPx: None

MoD: Caused by any disruption in the sympathetic chain (1st-order, 2nd-order, 3rd-order neuron) by stroke, Pancoast tumor (tumor at apex of lung), spinal cord hemisection, carotid dissection

- 1st-order neuron: Hypothalamus -(descending sympathetic chain)→ ciliospinal center of Budge (C8-T2)
- 2nd-order neuron: Ciliocenter of Budge → exit at T1 –(cervical sympathetic chain near lung apex)→ superior cervical ganglion
- 3rd-order neuron = two branches
- Branch 1: Superior cervical ganglion –(cavernous sinus, internal carotid artery)→ long ciliary nerve → pupillary dilator, superior tarsal muscle, sweat glands of forehead
- Branch 2: Superior cervical ganglion –(external carotid artery)→ sympathetic nerves to sweat glands of lower face

Dx:
1. Head CT to r/o cavernous sinus thrombosis
2. MRI to r/o stroke
3. CXR to r/o Pancoast tumor

Tx/Mgmt: Tx by etiology (i.e., stroke treatment, surgical removal of Pancoast tumor)

> **QUICK TIPS**
> Ptosis + Miosis + Anhidrosis* → Horner Syndrome. *Anhidrosis is an inconstant feature

Peripheral Nerve Injury and Disorders

This section deals with the peripheral nerve injuries outside of the cranial nerves. This is divided into 3 sections: (1) peripheral nerve disorders of upper extremity (UE), (2) peripheral nerve disorders of lower extremity (LE), (3) systemic peripheral nerve disorders.

Peripheral Nerve Disorders of Upper Extremity (Fig. 10.2)

A. Erb-Duchenne Palsy (Upper Trunk Lesion)

Buzz Words: Recently delivered infant + arm adducted, pronated, wrist flexed → Erb-Duchenne palsy (Fig. 10.3)
- Aka "Waiter's Tip" or "Bellman's" posture

Clinical Presentation: Erb-Duchenne palsy occurs in newborns and is also known as "Waiter's Tip" or

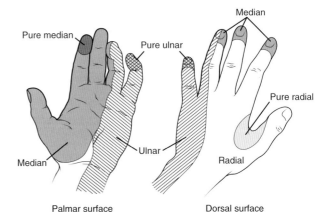

FIG. 10.2 Radial, median, ulnar nerve sensory distribution. (From Trott AT: *Wounds and lacerations*, ed 4. Philadelphia, 2012, Saunders.)

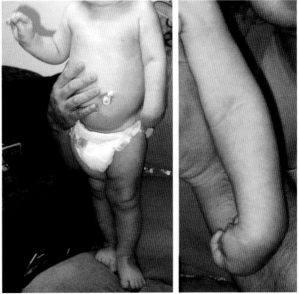

FIG. 10.3 Erb palsy. (From Graham JM, Sanchez-Lara PA: *Smith's recognizable patterns of human deformation*, ed 4. Philadelphia, 2016, Elsevier.)

"Bellman's" posture. Although anxiety-provoking for parents, this disorder is usually self-limited.

PPx: None

MoD: Traction on upper trunk (C5-C6) of brachial plexus → weakness of deltoid, biceps, infraspinatus, wrist extensors

Dx: Clinical

Tx/Mgmt: Conservative, self-resolving

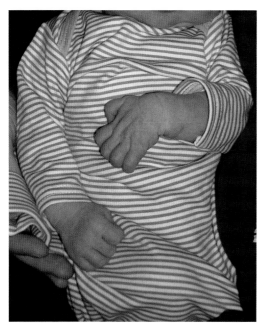

FIG. 10.4   Klumpke palsy. (From Buchanan EP, Richardson R, Tse R: Isolated lower brachial plexus (Klumpke) palsy with compound arm presentation: case report. *J Hand Surg Am.* 38(8):1567–1570, 2013.)

B. Klumpke Palsy (Brachial Plexus Lower Trunk Injury)

Buzz Words:
- Adult + grabbed branch during fall + atrophy of hypothenar muscles + sensory loss of pinky and lateral ring finger → Klumpke palsy 2/2 mechanical stress
- Recently delivered infant subject to upward force on arm during delivery → Klumpke palsy 2/2 birth trauma (Fig. 10.4)

Clinical Presentation: Be sure to identify the Buzz Words of Klumpke palsy and differentiate from Erb-Duchenne.

PPx: Avoid stretch-like motion

MoD: Traction on lower trunk (C8-T1) of brachial plexus → weakness of intrinsic hand muscles: lumbricals, interossei, thenar, hypothenar, sensory loss of ulnar distribution

Dx: Clinical exam

Tx/Mgmt: Conservative, self-resolving

C. Thoracic Outlet Syndrome

Buzz Words: Klumpke palsy + Horner syndrome + hoarseness

Clinical Presentation: Thoracic outlet syndrome occurs when the lower brachial plexus is compressed between the clavicle and first rib by some process, most commonly a Pancoast tumor.

99 AR

Pancoast Syndrome

PPx: None

MoD: Mass compressing lower trunk of brachial plexus between the clavicle and first rib

- Apical lung tumor most common → compresses sympathetic chain (Horner) + recurrent laryngeal nerve (hoarseness) + lower trunk of brachial plexus (Klumpke palsy)

Dx:

1. Electromyography (EMG)
2. X-ray (XR) to r/o lung tumor
3. CT

Tx/Mgmt:

1. Surgical decompression
2. Removal of tumor

D. Axillary Neuropathy

Buzz Words: Fracture of proximal humerus + inability to abduct shoulder + loss of sensation on lateral shoulder

Clinical Presentation: Commonly asked on the neurology and surgery shelf exams. Remember that the axillary nerve innervates the deltoid.

PPx: None

MoD: Fracture of proximal humerus or anterior dislocation of humerus → lesion of axillary nerve

Dx: XR of the proximal humerus

Tx/Mgmt:

1. Immobilization in sling
2. Analgesics
3. Orthopedic surgery for complex fractures

E. Musculocutaneous Neuropathy

Buzz Words: Loss of sensation on lateral forearm + weakness of biceps and supination + post-shoulder surgery

Clinical Presentation: Musculocutaneous neuropathy most frequently presents as numbness on lateral forearm. If you know that Buzz Word, you are almost guaranteed one correct answer on the neurology shelf.

PPx: None

MoD: Lesion of musculocutaneous nerve or upper trunk compression

Dx: XR of the cervical spine

Tx/Mgmt:

1. Supportive
2. Operative if complex fracture

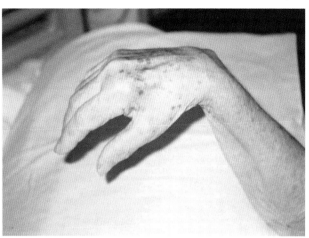

FIG. 10.5 Wrist drop. (From Bertorini TE: *Neuromuscular case studies*. Philadelphia, 2008, Butterworth-Heinemann.)

F. Brachial Plexitis (aka Parsonage-Turner Syndrome, aka Brachial Neuritis)

Buzz Words: Adult + burning shoulder/lateral neck pain + numbness/weakness of UE + resolves after 12 weeks

Clinical Presentation: Low-yield but can appear as distractor answer

PPx: None

MoD: Inflammation of brachial plexus—associated with diabetes, SLE, and polyarteritis nodosa, and may follow viral infections

Dx:

1. Cervical neck XR
2. Nerve conduction studies and EMG

Tx/Mgmt: Supportive, analgesics

G. Radial Neuropathy (aka Saturday Night Palsy)

Buzz Words:

- Crutch use/arm slung over park bench/fracture of spiral groove of humerus + wrist drop (Fig. 10.5) + sensory loss of dorsolateral hand → radial neuropathy
- Handcuffs + sensory loss of dorsolateral hand → cheiralgia paresthetica (aka handcuff neuropathy); occurs when only sensory branch of radial nerve is injured

Clinical Presentation: The most high-yield fact about radial neuropathy is that it is associated with a fracture of the spiral groove of the humerus.

PPx: Avoid compressing armpit/axilla

MoD: Compression of armpit or fracture (fx) of spiral groove of humerus → radial nerve damage

Dx: Arm and cervical XR

99 AR

| Cheiralgia Paresthetica |

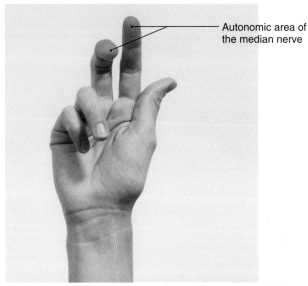

Autonomic area of the median nerve

FIG. 10.6 Pope's blessing. (From Paulsen F: *Sobotta Atlas of Human Anatomy*, ed 15. Munich, 2013, Elsevier GmbH.)

Tx/Mgmt:
1. If fracture, reduce and cast
2. If no fracture, supportive

H. Median Neuropathy

Buzz Words: Fracture of distal humerus or fx of distal radius + weakness of wrist flexion, abduction, opposition of thumb
  • Sign known as "Preacher's hand," "Ape hand," or "Pope's blessing" (Fig. 10.6)

Clinical Presentation: Median nerve neuropathy is associated with a fracture at the level of the distal humerus and distal radius.

PPx: Avoid fracture

MoD: Lesion of median nerve as it crosses distal humerus and distal radius

Dx: XR of arm, forearm

Tx/Mgmt:
1. Reduce fracture and cast
2. Supportive care

I. Carpal Tunnel Syndrome (CTS)

Buzz Words: Pregnant + hyper/hypothyroid + repetitive hand work + pain in wrist/hand at night + numbness/tingling of fingers + positive Phalen or Tinel sign

Clinical Presentation: Because CTS is so easy to recognize, the shelf frequently likes to test on the order of steps for both diagnosis and treatment. Make sure you know each step well and in order.

gg AR
Phalen Test

gg AR
Tinel Signs

gg AR
Carpal Tunnel Syndrome

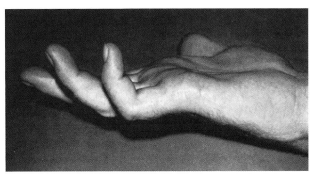

FIG. 10.7 Ulnar claw. (From Katirji B: Electromyography in clinical practice: a case study approach, St Louis, 1998, Mosby.)

PPx: Avoid repetitive wrist motion (e.g., extensive flexion and extension)

MoD: Compression of the median nerve 2/2 swelling, often in the fibromuscular groove posterior to the medial epicondyle of the humerus
- Can be 2/2 diabetes, hypo/hyperthyroidism, acromegaly, pregnancy, dialysis-related amyloidosis

Dx:
1. Clinical
2. Wrist XR to r/o fractures/arthritis
3. Nerve conduction studies are the most likely to confirm the diagnosis (per NBME)
4. Electromyography (if surgery is required)
5. CT/MRI only if EMG equivocal

Mgmt/Tx:
1. Rest
2. Splint
3. Nonsteroidal anti-inflammatory drugs (NSAIDs)
4. Corticosteroid shots (effective in 80%–90% of patients but may return after months; should not be given >3 times a year)
5. Surgery (carpal tunnel release) as last resort (must have EMG beforehand)

J Ulnar Neuropathy

Buzz Words: Fracture of medial epicondyle of elbow ("funny bone") + weakness of finger adduction/abduction, flexion of pinky/ring, wrist flexion/adduction + sensory loss of 4th/5th digit → ulnar neuropathy
- Sign known as "ulnar claw" (Fig. 10.7) or "benediction posture"

Clinical Presentation: Ulnar nerve neuropathy is associated with a fracture of the medial epicondyle of the elbow

PPx: None

MoD: Fracture of medial epicondyle of humerus → lesion of ulnar nerve

QUICK TIPS
Know the sequence of diagnostic and treatment steps! This is a common test question on the shelf (e.g., patient has already tried rest, splint, and NSAIDs. What is the next best treatment?)

QUICK TIPS
Differentiate from Klumpke palsy/thoracic outlet syndrome because there is no Horner syndrome or hoarseness.

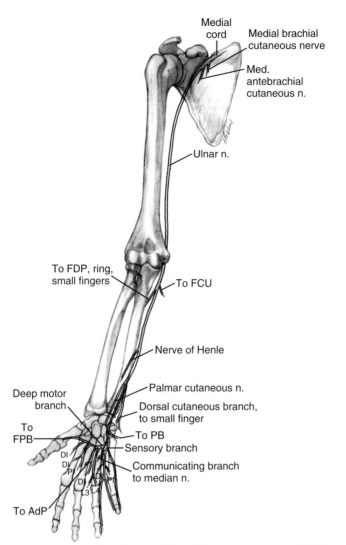

FIG. 10.8 Elbow and ulnar nerve. *AdP,* Adductor pollicis; *FCU,* flexor carpi ulnaris; *FDP,* flexor digitorum profundus; *FPB,* flexor pollicis brevis; *PB,* palmaris brevis. (From Doyle JR, Botte MJ: *Surgical anatomy of the hand and upper extremity.* Philadelphia, 2003, Lippincott Williams and Wilkins, p. 201; with permission.)

Dx: Arm XR

Tx/Mgmt:

1. Reduce fracture and splint
2. Supportive

K. Cubital Tunnel Syndrome

Buzz Words: Ulnar claw + sensory loss of ulnar distribution + history of prolonged pressure to medial elbow (i.e., leaning on table) (Fig. 10.8) → cubital tunnel syndrome

Clinical Presentation: If patient experiences ulnar neuropathy even if the patient does not have a history of acute injury, consider cubital tunnel syndrome, which occurs due to prolonged force.

PPx: Avoid compression of medial epicondyle

MoD: Compression of ulnar nerve at medial epicondyle of humerus from prolonged external force

Dx: Nerve conduction studies

Tx/Mgmt:

1. Splinting at night with elbow extended 45 degrees
2. Surgical decompression if conservative treatment fails

Peripheral Nerve Disorders of Lower Extremity (Fig. 10.9)

L. Femoral Neuropathy

Buzz Words: History of pelvic surgery + weakness of hip flexion/knee extension + loss of patellar reflex + sensory loss of anterior thigh

Clinical Presentation: Make sure to know the sensory distribution of the femoral nerve.

PPx: Avoid lesion during surgery

MoD: Lesion of femoral nerve during pelvic surgery, 2/2 retroperitoneal hematoma or pelvic mass

Dx: Physical exam

Tx/Mgmt:

1. Removal of mass if mass effect
2. Otherwise conservative management

M. Obturator Neuropathy

Buzz Words: Numbness of medial thigh + weakness with thigh adduction + history of surgery

Clinical Presentation: The obturator nerve supplies a small patch of skin with sensation on the medial thigh, but it is crucial in the functioning of muscles in the medial compartment of the thigh.

PPx: None

MoD: Lesion of obturator nerve

Dx: Physical exam

Tx/Mgmt:

1. Conservative
2. Decompressive surgery if mass effect present

N. Sciatic Neuropathy

Buzz Words: Posterior hip dislocation/IM injection to medial-inferior in buttock + loss of Achilles reflex + weakness of all foot/ankle muscles + sensory loss of foot/ankle

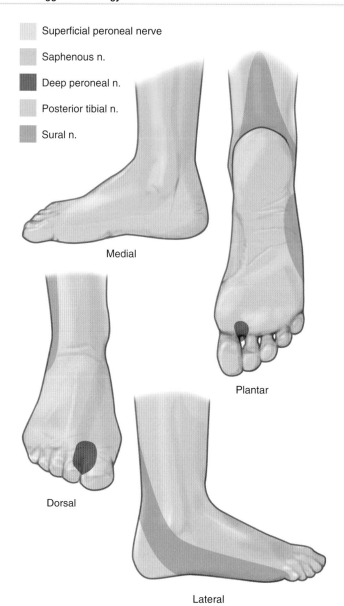

Superficial peroneal nerve

Saphenous n.

Deep peroneal n.

Posterior tibial n.

Sural n.

Medial

Plantar

Dorsal

Lateral

FIG. 10.9 Important nerves in the leg. (From Kadakia AR: Leg, Ankle, and Foot Diagnosis and Decision Making. In Miller MD, Thompson SR, editors: *DeLee & Drez's orthopaedic sports medicine*, ed 4. Philadelphia, 2015, Saunders.)

Clinical Presentation: Sciatic neuropathy frequently presents as leg pain that is worse than back pain. Sciatic neuropathy is not the same thing as "sciatica," which is a general term used to describe all painful disorders of sciatic distribution (and most commonly caused by compression of lumbosacral roots by slipped disc/osteophytes).

PPx: None
MoD: Lesion of sciatic nerve
Dx: Physical exam
Tx/Mgmt:
1. Treatment of etiology (e.g., reduction of posterior hip dislocation)
2. Supportive treatment

O. Common Peroneal Palsy
Buzz Words:
- Foot drop + inability to evert/dorsiflex foot + loss of sensation of foot and leg + injury to proximal lateral leg (fibula) → common peroneal palsy
- Foot drop + **loss of sensation between 1st/2nd toes** → deep peroneal nerve injury only
- Peroneal tunnel syndrome presents the same way, except for chronic (rather than acute) insult to proximal fibular head
- Weakness of plantar flexion + loss of sensation on dorsum of foot → superficial peroneal nerve injury only

Clinical Presentation: The most commonly tested concept is that a lesion to the deep peroneal nerve leads to loss of sensation in the web space between the first and second toes. This concept will likely show up at least once or twice on your shelf.
PPx: Avoid injury
MoD: Traumatic injury of common peroneal (or deep/ superficial peroneal) nerve; can also be 2/2 increased pressure of leg compartments
Dx:
1. Pressure measurement of leg compartments to r/o compartment syndrome
2. Repair of associated fx
3. Supportive
Tx/Mgmt: Treat based on etiology (i.e., surgery for compartment syndrome, reduction of fracture, etc.)

99 AR
Loss of sensation in web space between 1st and 2nd toe = deep peroneal nerve injury

P. Meralgia Paresthetica
Buzz Words: Sensory loss of lateral thigh + abdomen/pelvic surgery + pregnancy + obese + hard objects in pockets of tight jeans
Clinical Presentation: Meralgia paresthetica is the loss of sensation to the lateral thigh due to a lesion of the lateral femoral cutaneous nerve (LFCN). Clinically, a lesion to the LFCN is inconsequential to function, and

it is often a phenomenon seen in patients who undergo hip surgery.

PPx: Avoiding lesion of the LFCN

MoD: Lesion of the LFCN either by compression or surgical lesion as it travels under the inguinal ligament, tensor fascia lata

Dx: Physical exam

T/Mgmt: Supportive (often resolves spontaneously)

Q. Morton Metatarsalgia (aka Neuroma)

Buzz Words: Palpable neuroma between third and fourth toe + wearing **tight** high-heel shoes or pointed cowboy boots + prolonged activity that force toes together + pain on plantar aspect of foot between metatarsal heads

Clinical Presentation: Patients with Morton metatarsalgia present with a lump between the third and fourth toes. The best prevention for this phenomenon is wearing wide shoes.

PPx: Wear wide shoes

MoD: Inflammation of the common digital nerve at the third interspace between the third and fourth toes

Dx: Physical exam

Tx/Mgmt:
1. Analgesics
2. Wearing wider shoes
3. Surgical excision if needed

R. Tarsal Tunnel Syndrome

Buzz Words: Pain (burning/tingling) of plantar medial heel + pain still persists at rest (vs. plantar fasciitis) + compression of lateral malleoli + Tinel over tarsal tunnel

Clinical Presentation: See Buzz Words.

PPx: Avoid compression of lateral malleoli

MoD: Compression of lateral malleoli or excessive pronation of hind foot → compression of posterior tibial nerve as it crosses through

Dx:
1. Exam
2. Nerve conduction studies

Tx/Mgmt:
1. NSAIDs
2. Steroid injection
3. Orthotics
4. Surgery: tarsal tunnel release

gg AR

Posterior Tibial Nerve

QUICK TIPS

Tarsal tunnel syndrome is analogous to carpal tunnel syndrome. It involves compression of the posterior tibial nerve or its branches.

Systemic Peripheral Nerve Disorders of Upper Extremity

S. Guillain-Barré Syndrome (GBS, aka Acute Idiopathic Polyneuritis, Acute Inflammatory Demyelinating Polyradiculoneuropathy [AIDP])

Buzz Words: Ascending persistent paralysis + LMN signs only + preceding infection + preceding bloody diarrhea (campylobacter jejuni) + high protein, normal white blood cell count (WBC)/glucose on cerebrospinal fluid (CSF) analysis + autonomic dysfunction + < 2 months

Clinical Presentation: GBS is a high-yield topic because it can very easily be confused with other disease states that lead to paralysis. On the shelf, it is associated with infectious organisms such as *Campylobacter jejuni*.

PPx: None

MoD: Viral or bacterial (*C. jejuni* or *Vibrio cholera*) infx → autoimmune attack of peripheral myelin 2/2 molecular mimicry → endoneural inflammation and demyelination of peripheral nerves
- Vs. polio, which is 2/2 endomysial inflammation of nerve

Dx:
1. Physical exam
2. Electrodiagnostic testing
3. LP will show **albuminocytologic dissociation** (e.g., normal WBC + normal glucose + high protein)
4. Measure **forced vital capacity** (FVC) to determine need for intubation
5. Head MRI to r/o stroke

Tx/Mgmt:
1. Fluids
2. IVIG
3. Plasmapheresis
4. Respiratory support/intubation if FVC < 15 mL/kg

T. Chronic Inflammatory Demyelinating Polyradiculoneuropathy (CIDP)

Buzz Words: Ascending persistent paralysis + LMN signs only + preceding viral illness + preceding bloody diarrhea (*C. jejuni*) + high protein, normal WBC/glucose on CSF analysis + >2 months → CIDP

Clinical Presentation: CIDP is similar to GBS. The most important change is that paralysis for patients with CIDP has lasted at least 2 months.

PPx: None

MoD: Viral or bacterial (*C. jejuni* or *V. cholera*) infx → autoimmune attack of peripheral myelin 2/2 molecular mimicry → endoneural inflammation

Dx:
1. Electrodiagnostic testing
2. LP

Tx/Mgmt:
1. Supportive
2. Steroids (unlike GBS)
3. IVIG

U. Miller-Fisher Syndrome

Buzz Words: Ophthalmoplegia + ataxia + areflexia + ptosis + pupillary abnormalities + normal nerve conduction velocities (vs. abnormal conduction velocities in GBS) → Miller-Fisher syndrome

Clinical Presentation: Miller-Fisher syndrome is a variant of GBS and is similar to Bickerstaff encephalitis (which has hyperreflexia and encephalopathy).

PPx: None

MoD: Autoimmune antibodies against GQ1b (a ganglioside component of nerve, associated with oculomotor nerves)

Dx:
1. Nerve conduction studies
2. LP
3. Serology (anti-GQ1b antibody confirms diagnosis)

Tx/Mgmt:
1. Supportive
2. IVIG

V. Charcot-Marie-Tooth (CMT) disease (aka peroneal muscular atrophy, aka hereditary motor and sensory neuropathy)

Buzz Words: High-arched foot (pes cavus) and hammer toes + distal leg muscle weakness/atrophy + foot drop + loss of p/t and p/v + loss of deep tendon reflexes (DTRs) + frequent sprained ankles + difficulty running → CMT disease

Clinical Presentation: Patients with CMT have a history of diabetes or sensory loss of the extremities. The high-arched foot of CMT is also seen in Friedreich ataxia. Normal (Type II) or slow (Type I) nerve conductions depend on CMT type

PPx: None

MoD: 2/2 duplication of peripheral myelin protein-22 gene (PMP22) on chromosome 17, autosomal dominant inheritance, defective production of proteins involved in structure and functional or peripheral nerves or the myelin sheath

Dx: Nerve conduction studies
Tx/Mgmt:
1. Orthotics/bracing to correct foot drop
2. Physical therapy
3. Foot surgery to treat pes cavus deformity and hammer toes

W. Herpes Zoster (Shingles)
Buzz Words:
- Lancinating pain + rash and vesicles 2–3 days after initiation of pain + dermatomal distribution + unilateral → varicella zoster
- Ear pain + facial paralysis + vertigo + vesicles present on areas of pain → Ramsay Hunt syndrome (zoster of geniculate ganglion)
- Painful vesicles on tip of nose + vesicular eruption/pain around the eye + dermatomal distribution → ophthalmic herpes zoster 2/2 involvement of nasociliary branch of V1 of trigeminal nerve

Clinical Presentation: Presentation depends on which nerves are affected.
PPx: Zoster vaccine for adults ≥ 60 years old (y/o)
MoD: Herpes Zoster infection of peripheral nerves
Dx: Tzank test → multinucleate giant cells
Tx/Mgmt:
1. Antivirals (acyclovir, famciclovir, valacyclovir)
2. Analgesics (NSAIDs)

QUICK TIPS

Distinguishing Ramsay Hunt syndrome from Bell palsy: Bell palsy will not manifest with vesicles in the auditory canal and auricle.

Neuropathic Pain Syndromes

These neuropathic pain syndromes are mostly associated with psych conditions. The most commonly tested one, however, is trigeminal neuralgia, which is not associated with psych disorders. If you have one take-home point from Section 3, memorize the Buzz Words and treatment for trigeminal neuralgia, because this is something that is tested on multiple shelf exams.

A. Complex Regional Pain Syndrome (aka Reflex Sympathetic Dystrophy, aka Causalgia, aka Reflex Neurovascular Dystrophy)
Buzz Words:
- Pain without nerve distribution + worsens with stress + red skin + autonomic instability/sympathetic changes (hot/cold skin, dry/sweaty skin) + joint contractures + in s/o psychologic stress → complex regional pains syndrome

- Cold + cyanotic + moist extremity + exquisitely sensitive to pain + crush injury + refractor to analgesics → complex regional pain syndrome (aka causalgia, aka reflex sympathetic dystrophy)

Clinical Presentation: Complex regional pain syndrome is chronic neuropathic pain that unexpectedly persists after bone/soft tissue injury (type I) or nerve injury (type II)

PPx: Vitamin C

MoD: Unclear, but likely 2/2 inflammation, increase release of substance P, calcitonin gene-related peptide + increased peripheral nociceptor sensitization

- Usually follows an injury such as amputation, stroke, or fracture

Dx: Exam

Tx/Mgmt:

1. Sympathetic nerve block if sympathetic in origin
2. Psychiatric treatment (e.g., mirror therapy)
3. NSAIDs
4. Tricyclic antidepressants
5. Steroids, 960 transcutaneous electrical nerve stimulation (TENS)

B. Fibromyalgia

Buzz Words: <50 y/o + difficulty sleeping + joint/**muscle** tenderness **generalized** + specific **tender points** upon palpation + worse with stress + fatigue + cognitive disturbance + paresthesias

- Vs. polymyalgia rheumatica which is >50 y/o + joint pain + **no muscle involvement**

Clinical Presentation: Fibromyalgia is not considered a peripheral nerve disorder but is included here because it is part of the differentials.

PPx: None

MoD: Unknown

Dx:

1. Rheumatoid factor to r/o rheumatoid arthritis (RA), anti-dsDNA to r/o SLE
2. ESR to r/o dermatomyositis
3. Diagnosis based on clinical criteria

Tx/Mgmt:

1. Exercise, stretching, heat, massage
2. Stress management
3. TCA or SNRI or anticonvulsant, pregabalin, duloxetine, and milnacipran (the three Food and Drug Administration (FDA)-approved medicines for fibromyalgia)

C. Postherpetic Neuralgia

Buzz Words: Older adult + **constant** pain in a dermatomal distribution + history of vesicles in dermatomal distribution

Clinical Presentation: See Buzz Words

PPx: Zoster vaccine

MoD: Herpes zoster, aka shingles infection, at one nerve root → chronic pain; mechanism not totally understood

Dx: Exam

Tx/Mgmt:
1. Lidocaine patch
2. TCA, gabapentin, or pregabalin

D. Phantom Limb Pain

Buzz Words: Postamputation + pain in the area of amputated limb → phantom limb pain

Clinical Presentation: See Buzz Words

PPx:
1. Adequate control of preop and postop pain
2. preemptive epidural anesthesia

MoD: Unclear

Dx: History

Tx/Mgmt:
1. Analgesics (tramadol, opioids, TCAs)
2. Surgery (neurectomy, stump revision)
3. Psychiatric therapy (cognitive behavioral therapy [CBT], mirror therapy, biofeedback)

E. Thalamic Pain Syndrome (aka Dejerine-Roussy Syndrome, aka Central Pain Syndrome)

Buzz Words: Stroke to thalamic region (e.g., numbness of affected areas) + after resolution of symptoms, pain in the areas affected by thalamic stroke + **allodynia** (pain from stimulus that normally does not cause pain)

Clinical Presentation: On the shelf, suspect thalamic pain syndrome if patient reports unusual pain s/p stroke.

PPx: None

MoD: Damage to thalamus and potential posterior insular cortex of the temporal lobe

Dx: CT/MRI to locate lesion

Tx/Mgmt: Analgesics (tramadol, opioids, TCAs)

F. Trigeminal Neuralgia (aka Tic Douloureux)

Buzz Words: Sharp, severe shooting pain in face (episodes last seconds) + bolt of lightning + brought on by touch + unshaven side of face with pain → tic douloureux (trigeminal neuralgia)

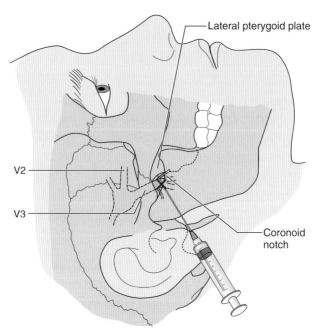

FIG. 10.10 Trigeminal neuralgia radiofrequency ablation. (From Waldman SD: Trigeminal nerve block: coronoid approach. In Waldman SD, editor: *Atlas of interventional pain management*, ed 2. Philadelphia, 2004, WB Saunders.)

PPx: None

MoD: Compression of trigeminal nerve by artery (i.e., AICA or ectatic basilar artery), vein or other mass

Dx: MRI to r/o organic causes

Tx/Mgmt:

1. Carbamazepine
2. Other meds like oxcarbazepine, gabapentin, baclofen, lamotrigine, amitriptyline
3. Radiofrequency ablation (Fig. 10.10)

GUNNER PRACTICE

1. A 42-year-old man comes to the physician because of a 2-week history of pain in the right side of the neck that radiates down the lateral aspect of the right arm to the third digit. He first noted the pain after lifting his 5-year-old son. He has also had mild weakness of the right arm in the right third digit. He works as a computer programmer, and spends most of his day at a keyboard. Examination shows mild weakness of right elbow and wrist extension, and a decreased right triceps reflex. Sensory examination shows no abnormalities. Which of the following is

the most likely location of the lesion causing this patient's symptom?
A. Basal ganglia
B. Brachial plexus
C. Cervical nerve root
D. Cervical spinal cord
E. Median nerve
F. Radial nerve
G. Thoracic nerve root
H. Ulnar nerve

2. A 63-year-old woman has been hospitalized for an allogeneic stem cell transplant for 7 weeks. She has been largely bed confined with multiple infections. She now complains of left leg weakness. Examination shows weakness of left ankle dorsiflexion, eversion, and great toe extension. There is decreased sensation on the dorsum of the left foot and anterolateral shin. Patellar, Achilles, brachioradialis, biceps, and triceps reflexes are 2+. What is the most likely diagnosis?
A. Common Peroneal neuropathy
B. Superficial Peroneal neuropathy
C. Lumbosacral plexitis
D. Tibial neuropathy
E. Deep Peroneal neuropathy
F. Femoral neuropathy
G. Obturator neuropathy

3. A 72-year-old man returns 5 weeks after triple coronary artery bypass surgery because of weakness of his left hand. He has pain along the medial aspect of his left hand and forearm that began immediately after the operation. He has weakness of left hand adduction and wrist flexion, thumb opposition, thumb abduction perpendicular to plane of palm, and finger abduction. What is the most likely diagnosis?
A. Median neuropathy
B. Ulnar neuropathy
C. Axillary neuropathy
D. Musculocutaneous neuropathy
E. Radial neuropathy
F. Brachial plexus injury

ANSWERS: What Would Gunner Jess/Jim Do?

1. WWGJD? A 42-year-old man comes to the physician because of a 2-week history of **pain in the right side of the neck that radiates down** the lateral aspect of the **right arm to the third digit.** He first noted the pain after lifting his 5-year-old son. He has also had mild weakness of the right arm in the right third digit. He works as a computer programmer, and spends most of his day at a keyboard. **Examination shows mild weakness of right elbow and wrist extension, and a decreased right triceps reflex. Sensory examination shows no abnormalities.** Which of the following is the **most likely location of the lesion** causing this patient's symptom?

Answer: C, Cervical nerve root

Explanation: This is the typical type of localization question one can expect on the shelf, particularly pertaining to peripheral nerve lesions. In particular, notice how the answer choices don't ask you to specify the nerve root, which would be a Step 1–level question. Instead, one can ascertain that this is a cervical spine problem due to the loss of only triceps reflex and weakness at level of elbow/wrist extension. This leaves cervical nerve root and spinal cord as the two remaining answer choices. Cervical spinal cord can be ruled out because there are no accompanying UMN lesions as one may expect from cervical myelopathy. Thus, cervical nerve root is the correct answer.

A. Basal ganglia → Incorrect. If a basal ganglia lesion, weakness and paralysis would be more widespread instead of localized. In addition, UMN signs like hyperreflexia would be present.

B. Brachial plexus → Incorrect. Brachial plexus includes all aspects of arm and hand movement and sensation. Thus if "sensory examination shows no abnormalities," meaning sensation is intact, the brachial plexus as a whole cannot be the location of the lesion.

D. Cervical spinal cord → Incorrect. A true cervical spinal cord injury would have signs below the level of the lesion, particularly UMN signs of the LE.

E. Median nerve → Incorrect. The median nerve is not responsible for the "triceps reflex" nor does it control "elbow and wrist extension."

F. Radial nerve → Incorrect. Although the radial nerve controls "elbow and wrist extension," it also contains sensory nerves. Thus it is not the best answer, since no sensory abnormalities are found. In general, a pure motor lesion localized to one area is traced back to a nerve root rather than the terminal branch.

G. Thoracic nerve root → Incorrect. Cervical nerve roots, specifically C7, control "triceps reflex" and wrist and elbow extension. Thoracic nerve roots are not involved.

H. Ulnar nerve → Incorrect. The ulnar nerve controls finger abduction/adduction, wrist flexion and adduction, which does not match the patient's deficits. Also, the ulnar nerve has sensory distributions as well, which would appear in an ulnar nerve lesion.

2. **WWGJD?** A 63-year-old woman has been hospitalized for an allogeneic stem cell transplant for 7 weeks. She has been largely bed confined with multiple infections. She now complains of left leg weakness. Examination shows weakness of left ankle dorsiflexion, eversion, and great toe extension. There is decreased sensation on the dorsum of the left foot and anterolateral shin. Patellar, Achilles, brachioradialis, biceps, and triceps reflexes are 2+. What is the most likely diagnosis?

Answer: A, Common peroneal neuropathy

Explanation: The common peroneal nerve first innervates the short head of the biceps femoris muscles before it divides into the superficial and deep peroneal nerves. The superficial peroneal nerve is very vulnerable to injury where it winds around the neck of the fibula, here affected by pressure from lying in bed and recent weight loss. If the common peroneal is injured, the foot cannot be everted or dorsiflexed. The deep peroneal innervates the tibialis anterior, extensor hallucis longus, and the extensor digitorum longus, which function to dorsiflex the foot and toe. The characteristic foot drop comes from a lesion of the deep peroneal nerve. Sensory changes with the deep peroneal nerve is in the region of the first interosseous space. Sensory changes when the superficial peroneal is involved go up over the dorsum of the foot sparing the lateral and medial borders and extend up along the anterolateral lag.

B. Superficial peroneal neuropathy → Incorrect. The motor and sensory deficits in this patient encompass more than just the superficial peroneal nerve; the motor and sensory deficits also affect the deep peroneal nerve.

C. Lumbosacral plexitis → Incorrect. If the patient had lumbosacral plexitis, the patient would experience more extensive motor and sensory deficits.

D. Tibial neuropathy → Incorrect. Patient does not have weakness of foot plantar flexion (weakness in gastrocnemius, soleus), or weakness of foot inversion (weakness of tibialis posterior), or the corresponding sensory deficits.

E. Deep peroneal neuropathy → Incorrect. The motor and sensory deficits in this patient encompass more than just the deep peroneal nerve; the motor and sensory deficits also affect the superficial peroneal nerve.

F. Femoral neuropathy → Incorrect. Patient does not have weakness of hip flexion (iliopsoas weakness) or weakness of knee extension (weakness of quadriceps), or the corresponding sensory deficits.

G. Obturator neuropathy → Incorrect. The patient does not have numbness of medial thigh or weakness with thigh adduction.

3. WWGJD? A 72-year-old man returns 5 weeks after triple coronary artery bypass surgery because of weakness of his left hand. He has pain along the medial aspect of his left hand and forearm that began immediately after the operation. He has weakness of left hand adduction and wrist flexion, thumb opposition, thumb abduction perpendicular to plane of palm, and finger abduction. What is most likely diagnosis?

Answer: F, Brachial plexus injury

Explanation: The patient was likely positioned incorrectly with the shoulder externally rotated and hyperabducted during the surgery, stretching the brachial plexus. To answer this question, it is important to figure out which nerves and muscles are involved in the aforementioned deficits. Hand adduction and wrist flexion are mediated by the flexor carpi ulnaris, thumb opposition is mediated by the opponens pollicis, thumb abduction perpendicular to the plane of the palm is mediated by the abductor pollicis brevis, and finger abduction is mediated by the dorsal interossei. The flexor carpi ulnaris and interossei are innervated by the ulnar nerve, and the opponens pollicis and the abductor pollicis brevis are innervated by the median nerve. Only a brachial plexus injury can account for lesions to both the median and ulnar nerves.

A. Median neuropathy → Incorrect. Although the patient has weakness of muscles innervated by the median nerve (opponens pollicis and abductor pollicis brevis), the patient also has weakness in muscles that are innervated by the ulnar nerve (flexor carpi ulnaris and interossei), which cannot be accounted for solely by median neuropathy.

B. Ulnar neuropathy → Incorrect. Although the patient has weakness of muscles innervated by the ulnar nerve (flexor carpi ulnaris and interossei), the patient also has weakness in muscles that are innervated by the median nerve (opponens pollicis and abductor pollicis brevis), which cannot be accounted for solely by ulnar neuropathy.

C. Axillary neuropathy → Incorrect. The patient does not have weakness of arm abduction at the shoulder, making axillary neuropathy unlikely.

D. Musculocutaneous neuropathy → Incorrect. The patient does not have weakness of elbow flexion, making musculocutaneous neuropathy unlikely.

E. Radial neuropathy → Incorrect. The patient does not have weakness of elbow extension, wrist extension, or finger extension, making radial neuropathy unlikely.

Vitamins and Drug Effects on the Nervous System

Leo Wang, Hao-Hua Wu, and Chuang-Kuo Wu

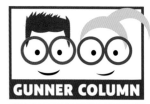

GUNNER COLUMN

Although there are many vitamins and associated disorders, your main task on the shelf is to identify the syndromes associated with deficiencies or toxicities. Prophylaxis (PPx) or treatment of these vitamin disorders are not high yield and easily generalized. The PPx to preventing any vitamin deficiency is a good healthy diet. The mechanisms for deficiency or toxicity of any of these diseases are beyond the scope of the shelf and reserved for Step 1; for the shelf, recognize the importance of vitamins in the major cellular metabolic processes.

The most important part of vitamin deficiencies is recognizing which clinical presentations are equivalent to which deficiencies and how specific vitamin deficiencies are obtained. Remember, vitamin deficiencies usually occur together, so don't be tricked if a particular patient doesn't fit into a cookie-cutter vitamin deficiency. They might have several. Typical diseases that do this are gastrointestinal (GI), but a non-GI cause of vitamin deficiency is cystic fibrosis. Lastly, making a diagnosis is straightforward by just recognizing the symptoms, although giving a trial of a vitamin to see if patients improve is also possible.

Vitamin Deficiencies

Of note, vitamin C deficiency is not covered in this section because no known neurologic sequelae result from not having enough vitamin C.

A. Vitamin A (Retinol) Deficiency
Buzz Words: Night blindness + dry skin + alopecia + corneal degeneration

Clinical Presentation: Vitamin A is a fat-soluble vitamin and requires pancreatic enzymes to be digested and absorbed. Thus it can be deficient in patients with pancreatic dysfunction or fat malabsorption.

PPx: Vitamin A supplementation

MoD: Lack of vitamin A, which is needed to bind a protein in retina, can cause inability to see through dim light at night (night blindness).

- Deficiency occurs rarely in fat malabsorption syndromes that are caused by cystic fibrosis, biliary atresia, and sprue.

Dx:
1. Clinical symptoms

Tx/Mgmt:
1. Vitamin A supplementation

B. Vitamin B1 (Thiamine) Deficiency

Buzz Words:
- Peripheral neuropathy with symmetric impairment of sensory, motor, and reflex functions → distal > proximal limb segments with calf muscle tenderness → dry beriberi
- Confusion + muscular atrophy + "edema" + tachycardia + cardiomegaly + CHF with peripheral neuropathy → wet beriberi
- Alcoholic with retrograde and anterograde amnesia and confabulation (altered mental status, ophthalmoplegia, ataxia [AOA]) → Wernicke-Korsakoff syndrome

Clinical Presentation: See Buzz Words

PPx: None; avoid abusing alcohol

MoD: Thiamine deficiency → catabolism of sugars and amino acids in neurons

Dx:
1. History and Physical

Tx/Mgmt:
1. Intravenous (IV) infusion of vitamin B1 in the acute stage (Wernicke encephalopathy). In the chronic stage (Korsakoff syndrome), only supportive care can be provided.

C. Vitamin B3 (Niacin; Nicotinic Acid) Deficiency

- aka Pellagra ("rough skin")

Buzz words: Diarrhea + dementia + dermatitis

Clinical Presentation: Very high yield. Patients with pellagra can present with a chief complaint of memory loss, dermatologic issues (e.g., dermatitis) or loose stools (diarrhea).

PPx: None

MoD: Decreased NAD production (NAD and its phosphorylated NADP form are cofactors required in many body processes); often from deficiency in tryptophan and occurring in people who consume only corn — lacking nicotinic acid and tryptophan that can be converted into nicotinic acid.
- Primarily causes symptoms of three organs (GI, nervous system, and skin)

QUICK TIPS
Beriberi means extreme weakness. The difference between dry and wet beriberi is whether or not edema of the lower extremities exists.

QUICK TIPS
Wernicke vs. Korsakoff: Wernicke = AOA, Korsakoff = confabulation

Dx:
1. Clinical syndrome—diarrhea, skin changes, and memory problem/inattention/confusion/spasticity

Tx/Mgmt:
1. Nicotinamide (same structure but lower toxicity)

D. Vitamin B6 (Pyridoxine) Deficiency

Buzz Words:
- Skin rash + atrophic glossitis with ulceration + angular cheilitis + conjunctivitis, intertrigo + neurologic symptoms of somnolence, confusion with sideroblastic anemia in patient with tuberculosis (TB) taking isoniazid therapy → B6 (pyridoxine) deficiency

Clinical Presentation: See Buzz Words. Can also present as seizures in an infant (pyridoxine-responsive seizure).

PPx: Vitamin supplementation with isoniazid for patients receiving TB treatment

MoD: Cofactor in reactions of amino acid, glucose, lipid metabolism → neuropathy from impaired sphingosine synthesis

Dx:
1. H&P (a. Seizures in infants, b. Neuropathy in adult patients)

Tx/Mgmt:
1. Pyridoxine hydrochloride to replace vitamin B6

E. Vitamin B12 (Cobalamin) Deficiency

Buzz words: Bone marrow promegaloblastosis (megaloblastic anemia from inhibition of purine synthesis) + GI symptoms + weakness + spasticity + absent reflexes + diminished vibration and position sensation + subacute degeneration of spinal cord + memory loss + depression → B12 deficiency

Clinical Presentation: Vitamin B12 deficiency is also known as subacute combined degeneration of the spinal cord that presents with posterior and lateral column signs.

PPx: B12 supplementation, diet including animal products

MoD: Decreased B12 → impaired DNA synthesis and regulation, fatty acid and amino acid metabolism

Dx:
1. Labs → vitamin B12 levels with elevated methylmalonic acid levels
2. Labs →anti-intrinsic factor antibodies to rule out (r/o) pernicious anemia

Tx/Mgmt:
1. Vitamin B12 supplementation

F. Vitamin D Deficiency

Buzz Words: Adult + Bone pain + weakness + poor fracture healing + hypocalcemic tetany

Clinical Presentation: Occurs in patients who do not have adequate exposure to sunlight.

PPx: Consumption of milk and sun exposure

MoD: Decreased vitamin D → decreased intestinal absorption of calcium and phosphate → decreased bone mineralization

Dx:
1. Serum level of 25-hydroxyvitamin D,
2. PTH levels to r/o endocrine disorder

Tx/Mgmt:
1. Vitamin D supplementation

G. Vitamin E Deficiency

Buzz Words: Hemolytic anemia + muscle weakness + acanthocytosis + spinocerebellar ataxia + loss of vibratory sensation and proprioception

Clinical Presentation: Cystic fibrosis patients can have vitamin E deficiency 2/2 pancreatic dysfunction.

PPx: None

MoD: Vitamin E protects cellular membranes and is an antioxidant

Dx:
1. H&P—ataxic gait and weakness in legs

Tx/Mgmt:
1. Supplementation with vitamin E

Adverse Drug Effects on the Nervous System

Psychotropic Drugs in the Nervous System

It is unlikely you will be tested on neuropsychiatric drugs on the neurology shelf, because these questions are more important for the psychiatry shelf. If you are asked, they will be as simple as recognizing overdose and withdrawal.

For the most part, you will want to know which psychiatric drugs are stimulants and which ones are depressants. When you withdraw, you always **do the opposite**. When you withdraw on a stimulant, you are depressed. When you withdraw on a depressant, you are stimulated. Effects of depression include lowered vital signs, whereas effects of stimulants include hyperactivity and increased vital signs. Examples of stimulants include amphetamines and cocaine. Examples of depressants include marijuana and opiates.

You should also recognize the hallucinogens because they tend to present more obviously: LSD, PCP, ketamine.

Nonpsychotropic Drugs in the Nervous System

A. Drug-Induced Meningitis

Buzz Words:
- Meningitis (fever, meningismus) in association with a new drug regimen of: nonsteroidal antiinflammatory drugs (NSAIDs), amoxicillin, azathioprine, methotrexate, IV immunoglobulin, isoniazid, allopurinol, lamotrigine, ranitidine, or sulfamethoxazole (Bactrim)

Clinical Presentation: See Buzz Words.

PPx: Avoid offending agents

MoD: Unknown most common—medicine overuse headache is caused by OTC NSAIDs

Dx:
1. H&P with med reconciliation,
2. LP/computed tomography/magnetic resonance imaging to rule out infectious cause

Tx/Mgmt:
1. Remove offending drug

B. Drug-Induced Neuropathy

The most commonly tested drugs that can cause neuropathy are vincristine and isoniazid. Being able to identify the side effects of these drugs are all that is required to answer relevant shelf questions.

Buzz Words:

Vincristine use (chemo regimen) + peripheral neuropathy + paralytic ileus → vincristine-induced neuropathy
- 2/2 inhibition of microtubule formation in nerve axons

TB patient or TB PPx + isoniazid use + hepatotoxicity + B6 deficiency → isoniazid-induced neuropathy
- 2/2 increased urinary excretion of pyridoxine and competition with vitamin B6 at neurotransmitters
- Isoniazid is structurally similar to vitamin B6

C. Drug-Induced Movement Disorders

Buzz Words:
- **Acute Dystonic Reaction:** 4 hours to 4 days, muscle spasm, stiffness, spasmodic torticollis, tongue protrusions, opisthotonus (hands/heels bend back, body bows forward), oculogyric crises (forced, sustained eye elevation)
- **Akathisia:** 4 days, motor restlessness

- **Parkinsonism:** 4 weeks, bradykinesia, shuffling gait, resting hand tremor
- **Neuroleptic Malignant Syndrome:** Within 7–10 days, but can happen anytime, hyperthermia, extreme rigidity, autonomic instability, "torticollis," elevated creatine kinase
- **Tardive Dyskinesia:** 4 months to 4 years, subtle, involuntary movements of tongue, face and extremities

Clinical Presentation: See Buzz Words.
PPx: Avoid antipsychotics (e.g., risperidone, haloperidol, etc.)
MoD: Due to dopamine's typical inhibitor effect in nigrostriatal pathway; in the absence of dopamine, there are extrapyramidal movement effects
Dx:
Clinical syndromes, as described in the previously.
Tx/Mgmt:

- Acute Dystonic Reaction: Anticholinergics (trihexyphenidyl/benztropine)
- Akathisia: Decrease drug, add propranolol
- Parkinsonism: Anticholinergics (trihexyphenidyl/benztropine)—DO NOT USE LEVODOPA
- Neuroleptic Malignant Syndrome: Supportive therapy, dantrolene last resort
- Tardive Dyskinesia: Replace whatever they were taking with clozapine

D. Serotonin Syndrome

Buzz Words: Hyperthermia + fever/tachycardia + rigidity + myoclonus + encephalopathy + diaphoresis
Clinical Presentation: Have a high suspicion for serotonin syndrome anytime patient has concomitant depression.
PPx: Avoid selective serotonin reuptake inhibitors
MoD: High levels of serotonin from using selective serotonin reuptake inhibitors (SSRIs) with monoamine oxidase inhibitors, illicit drugs, or herbal medications
Dx:
1. H&P
Tx/Mgmt:
1. Stopping the usage of the precipitating drugs,
2. Supportive care with control of agitation, autonomic instability, and hyperthermia,
3. Cyproheptadine (a serotonin 2A antagonist—antidote) for moderate to severe patients

> **MNEMONIC**
> Patients are **HARMED** by serotonin syndrome
> Hyperthermia, Autonomic instability, Rigidity, Myoclonus, Encephalopathy, Diaphoresis

GUNNER PRACTICE

1. A 35-year-old female presents to the emergency room with fever and difficulty with movement. She has a past medical history significant for depression and hypertension, which she is taking medications for. The patient's sister reports patient recently started taking a new drug for her "mood" but is not sure what. On exam, patient is sweating profusely and not oriented to time and location. She has a temperature of 104°F and a heart rate of 110 beats/min. What is the most appropriate treatment for this patient?
   A. Acetaminophen
   B. Paroxetine
   C. Cyproheptadine
   D. Ciprofloxacin
   E. Cetirizine

2. A 20-year-old male comes into the student health clinic with complaints of a strange "rash" on his chest. He also complains of frequent loose bowel movements and being more "forgetful" in class, which has affected his school performance. His past medical history is significant for a "kidney disease" that he cannot recall the name of. On exam, patient has a broad collar hyperpigmented rash that spans his collarbone. What is the most likely cause of his symptoms?
   A. Vitamin B1 deficiency
   B. Vitamin B3 deficiency
   C. Vitamin B6 deficiency
   D. Vitamin D deficiency
   E. Vitamin E deficiency

3. A homeless female of unknown age is brought into the emergency room by the police for "wandering around and acting crazy." On examination, patient has an **unsteady gait**, is slurring her words, and is oriented only to self. She was last admitted to the hospital 1 month ago for alcohol detox. What is the most appropriate next step in management?
   A. Thiamine supplementation
   B. Niacin supplementation
   C. Vitamin E supplementation
   D. Paroxetine
   E. Haloperidol

Notes

ANSWERS: What Would Gunner Jess/Jim Do?

1. WWGJD? A 35-year-old female presents to the emergency room with fever and difficulty with movement. She has a past medical history significant for depression and hypertension, which she is taking medications for. The patient's sister reports patient recently started taking a new drug for her "mood" but is not sure what. On exam, patient is sweating profusely and not oriented to time and location. She has a temperature of 104°F and a heart rate of 110 beats/min. What is the most appropriate treatment for this patient?

Answer: C, Cyproheptadine

Explanation: This patient has all the signs and symptoms of serotonin syndrome, Hyperthermia, Autonomic instability, Rigidity and Myoclonus (implied with difficulty of movement), Encephalopathy (A&Ox1) and Diaphoresis [HARMED]. Serotonin syndrome is treated with withdrawal of SSRIs and cyproheptadine. Acetaminophen would be used to reduce the fever but would not correct the underlying conduction.

    A. Acetaminophen → Incorrect. Although it can help to reduce the fever, acetaminophen does not treat the underlying condition

    B. Paroxetine → Incorrect. Another SSRI would only exacerbate the patient's symptoms

    D. Ciprofloxacin → Incorrect. Patient's fever is 2/2 due to an overload of serotonin and not due to an infection.

    E. Cetirizine → Incorrect. Patient does not have an allergy that needs to be treated.

2. WWGJD? A 20-year-old male comes into the student health clinic with complaints of a strange "rash" on his chest. He also complains of frequent loose bowel movements and being more "forgetful" in class, which has affected his school performance. His past medical history is significant for a "kidney disease" that he cannot recall the name of. On exam, patient has a broad collar hyperpigmented rash that spans his collarbone. What is the most likely cause of his symptoms?

Answer: B, Vitamin B3 deficiency

Explanation: Patient likely has niacin deficiency, aka pellagra, 2/2 Hartnup disease, a "kidney disease" in which neutral amino acids such as tryptophan are not properly reabsorbed. The classic presentation of pellagra is the 3 *Ds*: Dermatitis, Dementia, and Diarrhea, which the patient had. Treatment should be with niacin supplementation.

A. Vitamin B1 deficiency → Incorrect. B1 deficiency would instead lead to wet or dry beriberi as well as Wernicke-Korsakoff syndrome.

C. Vitamin B6 deficiency → Incorrect. B6 deficiency would instead present with atrophic glossitis, confusion, or somnolence, most commonly in the setting of concomitant isoniazid use.

D. Vitamin D deficiency → Incorrect. Vitamin D deficiency would lead to osteomalacia or tetany from abnormal levels of calcium.

E. Vitamin E deficiency → Incorrect. Vitamin E deficiency would lead to other symptoms such as spinocerebellar ataxia and hemolytic anemia.

3. WWGJD? A homeless female of unknown age is brought into the emergency room by the police for "wandering around and acting crazy." On examination, patient has an unsteady gait, is slurring her words, and is oriented only to self. She was last admitted to the hospital 1 month ago for alcohol detox. What is the most appropriate next step in management?

Answer: A, thiamine supplementation

Explanation: The patient clearly has two of the three symptoms associated with vitamin B1 (thiamine) deficiency: altered mental status and ataxia. The third symptom is typical ophthalmoplegia. Patients suspected of alcohol abuse who present with intoxication are routinely given thiamine to treat or prevent the development of further symptoms. Failure of treatment and chronic alcohol abuse may lead to Korsakoff syndrome, which is characterized by damage to the mammillary bodies and confabulation.

B. Niacin supplementation → Incorrect. Acute alcohol intoxication leads to thiamine and not niacin deficiency.

C. Vitamin E supplementation → Incorrect. Vitamin E deficiency is not associated with alcohol abuse.

D. Paroxetine → Incorrect. SSRIs are never appropriate for acute management of patients as they take at least several weeks before taking effect. The patient in this question stem also does not have a disorder treatable with an SSRI.

E. Haloperidol → Incorrect. Although haloperidol is often administered as a way to calm patients, the patient in this question stem is not being disruptive. In addition, antipsychotics are not part of the acute alcohol intoxication management pathway.

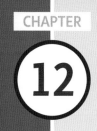

CHAPTER

12

Metabolic Disorders on the Neurology Shelf

Catherine Blebea, Hao-Hua Wu, Leo Wang, and Chuang-Kuo Wu

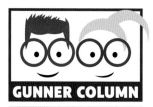

GUNNER COLUMN

Metabolic disorders of neurology are disorders that do not directly affect neurologic structures. Instead, defects in metabolism indirectly affect neurologic structures through chemical mediators, such as toxic metabolites. For example, in hepatic encephalopathy, a syndrome where abnormal metabolites from hepatic failure alter the activity of the central nervous system, excess ammonia can cross the blood-brain barrier from the blood supply and can influence neurologic function. Because of how rare some of these neurologic metabolic disorders are, this is not a commonly tested topic of the shelf. However, you should still be very familiar with disease processes like hepatic encephalopathy and Wilson disease because they have broad signs and symptoms spanning multiple disciplines such as medicine, psychiatry, and pediatrics.

Metabolic Disorders

A. Adrenoleukodystrophy (aka X-linked Adrenoleukodystrophy, X-ALD, ALD)

Buzz Words:

- Adrenal insufficiency is the only symptom → Addison disease
- Elevation of very long chain fatty acid (VLCFA) + male in 30s–50s + spastic paraplegia *(progressive weakness and stiffness in the lower limbs)* to paraparesis *(paralysis of lower limbs)* + impotence + Addison disease + gate disturbances → adrenomyeloneuropathy (AMN)
- Elevation of VLCFA + 4–8-year-old male + vision and hearing impairments + progressive motor deficits + seizures + rapid neurologic and cognitive decline to death/total impairment 2–4 years after onset → cerebral demyelinating form of ALD

Clinical Presentation: The most high-yield fact in this section is the treatment of X-ALD with Lorenzo's oil. The rest of the sections are low yield.

PPx: None

MoD: X-linked disease that affects the peroxisomes

Deficiency of the peroxisomal membrane transporter adrenoleukodystrophy protein (ALDP), which is encoded on the X chromosome. ALDP disrupts VLCFA metabolism and causes a buildup of VLCFA in the nervous system, testes, and adrenals.

> **MNEMONIC**
>
> A key distinction between AMN and the cerebral form is the age of onset.
>
> AMN: adults
> Cerebral form: children
> Although AMN can progress to the cerebral form, this is rare.

> **QUICK TIPS**
>
> Don't memorize genetic details for the shelf. However, you may score bonus points with your attending for knowing that the ALDP protein is encoded by the gene ABCD1.

Dx:
1. Look for elevated VLCFA in serum, can confirm diagnosis with genetic testing.

Tx/Mgmt:
1. Lorenzo's oil, a 4:1 mixture of oleic acid and erucic acid, and reduced fat intake to lower plasma VLCFA levels is recommended. If adrenal insufficiency is present (seen in ⅔ of patients), patients should receive adrenal replacement therapy.

gg AR

Lorenzo's oil was discovered by the father of a child with ALD who was frustrated by the lack of medical treatment for ALD.

B. Metabolic Encephalopathy

Metabolic encephalopathies are neurologic disorders **NOT** caused by structural abnormalities but instead result from other illnesses. Common diseases that can cause metabolic encephalopathy include diabetes, liver disease, renal failure, and heart failure. Therefore the encephalopathy is generally **reversible** if systemic disorder is treated. Although they all have decreased cerebral function as a symptom, the mechanism of disease, symptoms, diagnosis, prophylaxis, and treatment/management will generally depend on the etiology.

Some Common Causes of Metabolic Encephalopathy

A. Hepatic Encephalopathy

Buzz Words: Altered consciousness or defects in cognition + asterixis *(flapping tremor of hands)* + history of alcohol abuse/signs of liver failure or cirrhosis

Clinical Presentation: Typically occurs in patients with a history of chronic alcohol abuse and will present as asterixis

PPx: Lactulose

MoD: Hyperammonemia → ammonia increases GABAergic neurotransmission in the brain → suppression of neuronal activity

gg AR

Example of asterixis

Dx:
1. Assume hepatic encephalopathy if there's evidence of significant liver disease or failure with altered cognition without another proven cause

Tx/Mgmt:
1. Treat first with lactulose, which inhibits ammonia production. If an alternative is needed, treat with rifaximin, which reduces ammonia-producing bacteria.

B. Hypoglycemic Encephalopathy

Buzz Words: Altered consciousness + severe hypoglycemia + seizures/muscle spasms + coma/death

Clinical Presentation: Patient presents with encephalopathic signs/symptoms in the setting of low blood sugar

PPx: Ensure appropriate blood glucose levels.

MoD: Low blood glucose → depletion of ATP in the brain→ abnormal neurologic function

Dx:

1. Evidence of abnormal mental status and a blood glucose level below 50 mg/dL

Tx/Mgmt:

1. Treat by administering glucose.

C. Uremic Encephalopathy

Buzz Words: Altered consciousness or confusion + seizures + asterixis + renal failure + coma → uremic/dialysis encephalopathy

Clinical Presentation: You may see in a question that a patient with suspected uremic encephalopathy had their cerebrospinal fluid (CSF) examined. In general, the CSF is abnormal and has high protein levels, although a normal CSF does not rule out uremic encephalopathy.

PPx: None

MoD: Renal failure leads to an increase in metabolites and hormones in the blood; these affect neurotransmitters in the brain, causing encephalopathy.

Dx: Assume uremic encephalopathy if there's evidence of significant renal disease or failure with altered cognition without another proven cause.

Tx/Mgmt: Treat with dialysis. If dialysis is insufficient, perform a renal transplant.

D. Wilson Disease

Buzz Words: Kayser-Fleischer ring on slit lamp *(copper buildup in cornea, appears to be a ring around the iris)* + seizures + hepatitis + involuntary muscle contractions (ataxia, dystonia) + low ceruloplasmin + high urine copper + "wing-beating" tremor → Wilson disease

Clinical Presentation: Wilson disease is the most high-yield disease of this chapter. Make sure to know the Buzz Words and the order of the diagnostic steps and treatment.

PPx: Chelation with penicillamine is the optimal prophylaxis. Alternative options include trientine or zinc.

MoD: Caused by an autosomal recessive mutation in an ATPase that transfers copper. Copper builds up primarily in the liver and brain.

Dx:

1. Gold standard: liver biopsy and copper testing.
   - A Kayser-Fleischer ring on slit lamp can be also used to make a definitive diagnosis.
   - Wilson disease is associated with low serum ceruloplasmin levels and high urine copper levels, but their absence does not rule out Wilson disease, and

99 AR

Kayser-Fleischer rings are the most important diagnostic sign of Wilson disease.

this method should be the lowest in importance for testing for Wilson disease.

Tx/Mgmt:

1. Lifelong chelation with penicillamine is the optimal treatment.

Alternative options include chelation with trientine or zinc. Liver transplant is recommended only for patients with extensive liver failure.

99 AR

"Wing-beating" tremors are a classic sign of Wilson disease.

GUNNER PRACTICE

1. A 63-year-old man is admitted to the hospital for a lumbar laminectomy. One day postoperatively, he has a low-grade fever secondary to a urinary tract infection. He also has difficulty sleeping at night, and treatment with lorazepam is started. Two days postoperatively, he becomes drowsy and confused. On examination, he is difficult to arouse and his speech is slurred. He is able to answer a few simple questions, but he thinks he is at home and the year is 1956. He cooperates poorly with formal strength testing. The remainder of the examination shows no abnormalities. Which of the following is the most likely diagnosis?
   A. Cerebral infarction
   B. Dementia, Alzheimer type
   C. Metabolic encephalopathy
   D. Nonconvulsive status epilepticus
   E. Subdural hematoma

2. A 75-year-old woman is admitted to the hospital for an acute onset of lethargy and confusion. She complains that she cannot draw complex figures, and she does not know the day of the week, month, or year. On physical exam, she has splenomegaly, hepatomegaly, and a positive fluid wave test. She admits to drinking five or six glasses of scotch per day for the past 34 years, and her past history is significant for hepatitis C infection. What should you do next?
   A. Test her blood ammonia levels
   B. Test her serum albumin
   C. Prescribe lactulose
   D. Arrange for a liver transplant
   E. Test for hepatitis C antibodies

3. An 18-year-old male presents to your clinic with seizures and dystonia. On physical exam, you notice he has a "wing-beating" tremor. You also notice copper deposits in the cornea. What is the best initial treatment for this patient?
   A. Chelation with penicillamine
   B. Chelation with zinc
   C. Liver transplant
   D. Chelation with trientine
   E. Start the patient on dialysis

ANSWERS: What Would Gunner Jess/Jim Do?

1. WWGJD? A 63-year-old man is admitted to the hospital for a lumbar laminectomy. One day postoperatively, he has a low-grade fever secondary to a urinary tract infection. He also has difficulty sleeping at night, and treatment with lorazepam is started. Two days postoperatively, he becomes drowsy and confused. On examination, he is difficult to arouse and his speech is slurred. He is able to answer a few simple questions, but he thinks he is at home and the year is 1956. He cooperates poorly with formal strength testing. The remainder of the examination shows no abnormalities. Which of the following is the most likely diagnosis?

Answer: C, Metabolic encephalopathy

Explanation: This question is answered through process of elimination and understanding the definition of metabolic encephalopathy, which is a **reversible** neurologic disorder caused by systemic illness. It is unlikely a structural lesion because his symptoms are all very nonspecific. For instance, the strength testing is noted as "cooperates poorly." This suggests that patient's strength is intact; it's just not able to be demonstrated through alteration of sensorium. The biggest clue is that the patient has "**no physical exam abnormalities.**" No sensory loss, no areflexia/hyperreflexia, no Babinski sign present (all of which are inferred by the aforementioned statement). Thus one can rule out structural diseases such as cerebral infarction (A), dementia (B), and subdural hematoma (E). This leaves metabolic encephalopathy and status epilepticus. The latter can be ruled out because patient can still "answer a few simple questions," which should not be the case if in the midst of a seizure. In addition, lack of any stereotypical convulsive movements rules out possibility that patient is suffering from postictal confusion (which is not even listed as an answer choice). Thus metabolic encephalopathy, likely sepsis from UTI, is the correct answer.

A. Cerebral infarction → Incorrect. As explained previously, there are no physical exam abnormalities, which makes structural lesions unlikely.

B. Dementia, Alzheimer type → Incorrect. In addition to the patient not suffering from a structural lesion, the patient's symptoms arise **acutely.** Dementia, Alzheimer type is a disease process that develops progressively over years, making this answer choice unlikely.

D. Nonconvulsive status epilepticus → Incorrect. As mentioned previously, the patient is able to answer questions in the middle of his episode of drowsiness/confusion, which is not something that happens in nonconvulsive status epilepticus.

E. Subdural hematoma → Incorrect. Similar to the explanation for answer choice (A), no physical exam findings imply that a structural lesion like a subdural hematoma would be unlikely.

2. WWGJD? A 75-year-old woman is admitted to the hospital for an acute onset of lethargy and confusion. She complains that she cannot draw complex figures, and she does not know the day of the week, month, or year. On physical exam, she has splenomegaly, hepatomegaly, and a positive fluid wave test. She admits to drinking five or six glasses of scotch per day for the past 34 years, and her past history is significant for hepatitis C infection. What should you do next?

Answer: C, Prescribe lactulose

Explanation: The patient's splenomegaly, hepatomegaly, and ascites as well as her history of alcoholism and hepatitis C indicate liver dysfunction. Her lethargy, lack of fine motor movements, and disorientation indicate cognitive impairment. The most likely diagnosis for her symptoms without an alternative explanation for her altered consciousness is hepatic encephalopathy. The treatment for hepatic encephalopathy is lactulose.

A. Test her blood ammonia levels. → Incorrect. You should already suspect hepatic encephalopathy, and the diagnosis of hepatic encephalopathy is independent of blood ammonia levels, despite ammonia's role in the mechanism of disease. The treatment is also not dependent on blood ammonia levels.

B. Test her serum albumin. → Incorrect. There is already clear evidence of liver disease, and the patient's history indicates that this is an acute process, so liver function tests are not necessary. Normal serum albumin also does not rule out liver dysfunction.

D. Arrange for a liver transplant. → Incorrect. With lactulose the patient's hepatic encephalopathy should resolve within 72 hours.

E. Test for hepatitis C antibodies. → Incorrect. It is not necessary to test for antibodies to hepatitis C as the patient already has a documented history of hepatitis C and therefore would have antibodies.

3. WWGJD? An 18-year-old male presents to your clinic with **seizures** and **dystonia.** On physical exam, you

notice he has a **"wing-beating" tremor.** You also notice copper deposits in a ring in the cornea. What is the best treatment for this patient?

Answer: A, Chelation with penicillamine

Explanation: This patient has Wilson disease, as evidenced by the Kayser-Fleischer rings and "wing-beating" tremor. Although the question does not specifically describe the copper rings as Kayser-Fleischer rings, you should be able to recognize them from the description. Kayser-Fleischer rings are traditionally examined with a slit lamp but can sometimes be seen with an unaided eye. The involuntary muscle contractions and seizures are also consistent with Wilson disease. The optimal treatment for Wilson disease is chelation with penicillamine.

B. Chelation with zinc. → Incorrect. Although this is a treatment for Wilson disease, chelation with penicillamine is preferred.

C. Liver transplant. → Incorrect. This patient does not exhibit any signs of severe liver dysfunction and therefore does not require a transplant.

D. Chelation with trientine. → Incorrect. Although this is a treatment for Wilson disease, chelation with penicillamine is preferred.

E. Start the patient on dialysis. → Incorrect. This patient does not exhibit any signs of severe liver dysfunction and therefore does not require a transplant.

Notes

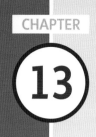

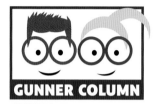

CHAPTER

13

Degenerative and Global Cerebral Dysfunction Disorders

Michael Baer, Hao-Hua Wu, Leo Wang, and Chuang-Kuo Wu

The focus of this chapter is on disorders that affect one or more areas of cognitive functioning. All of the disorders covered in the degenerative and global cerebral dysfunction section lead to momentary or permanent cognitive impairments.

This chapter is divided into two main sections. First, degenerative neurologic disorders will be discussed. These disorders are characterized by a gradual onset and progressive, irreversible decline in cognitive function, and include Alzheimer disease, dementia with Lewy bodies, frontotemporal dementia, and Huntington disease (HD). These important disorders are often tested on the neuro shelf, psychiatry shelf, and the medicine shelf, so their presentations and causes are important to learn.

The second section discusses the global cerebral dysfunction disorders. These disorders are often brought up as answer choices, so it is important to recognize common disease buzz words, such as sundowning for delirium and transient loss of memory/ability to learn in transient global amnesia.

Degenerative Neurologic Disorders

The degenerative neurologic disorders predominantly refer to diseases that lead to dementia—i.e., a progressive decline in cognition, language, memory, or personality. Although there is significant overlap in the clinical presentation of dementias, the presenting symptoms may offer clues to the underlying cause. Alzheimer disease tends to first cause memory loss, frontotemporal dementia initially causes personality changes, and Lewy body dementia (LBD) exhibits Parkinsonian signs. The clinical presentations often correspond to the brain regions most impacted by disease (i.e., frontotemporal dementia will show changes in behavior and dramatic atrophy of the frontal lobes). For most degenerative neurologic disorders, the underlying pathology is based on the accumulation and spread of abnormally folded proteins, such as beta amyloid plaques and abnormal tau protein phosphorylation in Alzheimer disease.

Although the dementias that result from degenerative neurologic disorders are irreversible, a similar clinical picture can result from reversible causes (dementia due to treatable conditions). The most commonly tested reversible causes of dementia include hypothyroidism, neurosyphilis, vitamin B12 deficiency, depression (pseudodementia), Wernicke-Korsakoff (alcohol related), normal pressure hydrocephalus, and infectious etiologies (like *Cryptococcus* and Lyme disease) (Table 13.1). A common workup to exclude reversible causes of dementia includes a computed tomography/magnetic resonance imaging (CT/MRI), lumbar puncture, rapid plasma reagin (RPR) for syphilis, and vitamin B12 and thyroid-stimulating hormone (TSH) levels. Screening for human immunodeficiency virus (HIV) and measurement of copper levels (Wilson disease), cortisol (Cushing disease), and heavy metal concentrations may be warranted with the appropriate clinical history. These diseases are covered in more detail elsewhere, but are worth reviewing while answering the questions found at the end of the chapter.

The degenerative neurologic diseases are organized based on their most common presenting symptom (Table 13.2). Because the presenting symptoms relate to the underlying pathology and distribution of disease, this approach provides a framework for organizing the different diseases during study.

Memory Loss as the Predominant Symptom

A. Alzheimer Disease

Buzz Words: Older individual + progressive forgetfulness + chronic and progressive + <24 on Mini-Mental State

QUICK TIPS
Dementia = persistent/progressive decline in intellectual/cognitive function with preserved consciousness

99 AR
Organizing Chart for Dementias

99 AR
Radiological Correlates of Dementia

QUICK TIPS
Dementia must be distinguished from age associated cognitive decline (small memory impairment that does not interfere with daily functioning)!

TABLE 13.1 Common Reversible Causes of Dementia

Metabolic	Infection/ inflammation	Structural	Others
Hypothyroidism	Meningitis	Subdural hematoma	Depression
Vitamin deficiencies (i.e., B12 and folate)	Encephalitis (HIV, herpes)	Normal pressure hydrocephalus	Polypharmacy
Liver failure	Neurosyphilis	Tumor	Alcohol abuse
Wilson disease	Lyme disease		Heavy metal exposure
Cushing disease	Sarcoidosis		
Prolonged hypoglycemia/ hypoxia			

HIV, Human immunodeficiency virus.

Examination (MMSE) + apraxia + aphasia + agnosia + impairs activities of daily living (ADLs) (vs. mild cognitive impairment or normal aging)

Clinical Presentation: Patients with Alzheimer disease are typically older than 60 years and present with reduction in short-term memory (unable to remember newly learned facts) and word-finding difficulty. Paranoia, personality changes, and executive dysfunction may also be prominent. Women are affected 3 times more often men. If there is Down syndrome in past medical history, symptoms will present much earlier in the patient's lifespan.

PPx: None

MoD:

- Mediated by amyloid beta plaques (extracellular) and neurofibrillary tangles (intracellular)
- Widespread neuronal loss and atrophy, prominent in the temporal lobe and extending to the frontal lobes, parietal lobes, the nucleus basalis of Meynert (cholinergic, see later for therapeutic implications)
- Down syndrome increases the risk of developing Alzheimer disease (because amyloid beta protein precursor is located on chromosome 21)

Gross Pathology of Alzheimer Disease

Effects of Plaques and Tangles in Alzheimer Disease

TABLE 13.2 Organizing chart for Neurodegenerative Conditions

Disease	Protein	Brain region affected	Predominant clinical features
AD	Beta-amyloid + Tau	Diffuse, prominent temporal atrophy	Memory loss
FTLD	Tau or TDP-43	Frontal/temporal lobes	Personality change/aphasias
PSP	Tau	Midbrain	Vertical gaze palsy
Parkinson	Alpha synuclein	Substantia nigra	Bradykinesia, resting tremor, postural instability, rigidity
DLB	Alpha synuclein	Cortex and substantia nigra	Dementia with Parkinson signs
HD	Polyglutamine expanded protein	Caudate and putamen	Chorea

AD, Alzheimer disease; *DLB*: dementia with Lewy bodies; *FTLD*, frontotemporal lobar degeneration; *HD*, Huntington disease; *PSP*, progressive supranuclear palsy.

- Familial types: mutations of genes of APP and pre-senilin-1 protein (PSEN-1) and presenilin-2 protein (PSEN-2) that can lead to abnormal amyloid peptide accumulation

Dx:

1. MMSE
2. Rule out (r/o) reversible causes of dementia by looking at TSH, T3, T4 or B12 levels, RPR for syphilis
3. Head MRI to r/o structural lesions, will show diffuse atrophy/enlarged ventricles with disproportionate atro-phy of the hippocampus
   - NOTE: As with the other neurodegenerative causes of dementia, the diagnosis cannot be definitive un-less an autopsy is performed.

Tx/Mgmt:

1. Donepezil (acetylcholinesterase [AchE] inhibitor)
2. Galantamine, rivastigmine (AChE inhibitors)
3. For moderate or severe → Memantine (N-methyl-D-aspartate [NMDA] antagonist)
   - Antipsychotics, such as Olanzapine and quetiapine, are sometimes used to control psychosis, aggres-sion, and agitation that may develop.

Behavioral and Personality Changes as the Predominant Symptom

A. Frontotemporal Dementia (FTLD, aka Pick Disease)

Buzz Words: Inappropriate behavior/poor judgment + personality changes + disinhibition + hypersexuality + snout reflex + intraneuronal silver staining inclusions (tau bodies aka Pick bodies) or TDP-43 inclusions

Clinical Presentation: Frontal temporal dementia is the second most common cause of early onset dementia (after Alzheimer disease). On the shelf, it can be identi-fied as a patient with memory difficulties who is disin-hibited (e.g., says things that are uncharacteristically offensive). It presents in patients older than 55 years of age with the chief complaint being one of two variants: behavioral and language.

Behavioral variant = personality changes predominate, apathy, disinhibition, perseveration, eating disor-ders, insight is impaired

Language variant = aphasias and apraxias are pre-dominant early symptoms

A significant number of FTLD patients will also have signs of motor neuron disease (amyotrophic lateral sclero-sis [ALS] is also caused by TDP-43 inclusions).

PPx: None

QUICK TIPS

Pick disease refers to a specific type of inclusion formed by the tau protein. While Pick disease is sometimes used to refer to FTLD in general, FTLD can also be formed by inclusions of a different protein (TDP-43).

AR

Neuropathological findings of FTLD

MoD: Severe atrophy of the frontal and temporal lobes secondary to:
- Tau protein inclusions OR
- TDP-43 protein inclusions

Dx:
1. MMSE, neurobehavioral assessment
2. CT/MRI → show disproportionate atrophy of frontal/temporal lobes
3. R/o reversible dementia (thyroid, B12)
   - NOTE: As with the other neurodegenerative causes of dementia, the diagnosis cannot be definitive unless an autopsy is performed.

Tx/Mgmt:
Only symptomatic treatment is currently available (no Food and Drug Administration approved drug)
- Olanzapine/antipsychotic for severe disinhibition, aggression, and agitation

Movement Disorder as the Predominant Symptom

A. Lewy Body Dementia

Buzz Words: Lilliputian hallucinations (benign hallucinations) + episodic confusion + impaired visuospatial function + dementia <12 months after onset of bradykinesia, tremor, abnormal posture, rigidity
- If >12 months, Parkinson disease (PD) with dementia (see below)

Clinical Presentation: LBD is high-yield because of its distinct Buzz Words in the setting of memory loss (e.g., Lilliputian hallucinations). If dementia >12 months, PD with dementia (see below). Patients present with Parkinsonian symptoms (bradykinesia, tremor, abnormal posture, rigidity) and dementia (dementia may precede or follow Parkinsonian symptoms)
- Visual hallucinations and REM sleep behavior disorders are often seen.

PPx: None

MoD: Intracytoplasmic alpha-synuclein inclusions diffusely seen throughout the cortex and substantia nigra; leads to degeneration of dopamine releasing neurons

Dx:
1. Clinical exam and history demonstrating Parkinsonian syndrome, recurrent hallucinations, REM sleep behavior disorders, and dementia
   - One clue to diagnosis is extreme sensitivity to neuroleptics—confusion, neuroleptic malignant syndrome, worsening Parkinson symptoms

QUICK TIPS

If a patient has hallucinations/paranoid delusions/episodic confusion early in the disease course, think Lewy Body Dementia. These are NOT common early in Alzheimers/FTLD.

QUICK TIPS

Neuroleptics = term for older typical antipsychotic drugs, such as haloperidol

Tx/Mgmt:
1. Treat Parkinsonian features with levo-carbidopa (but may lead to worsening hallucinations/delirium)
2. Treat cognitive symptoms with acetylcholinesterase inhibitors (Donepezil)
   - Dopaminergic agonists often trigger visual hallucinations and psychotic behaviors.
   - Hypersensitivity to antipsychotics.

B. Parkinson Disease

Buzz Words: Cogwheel rigidity + resting tremor + shuffling gait + akinesia + dementia after 12 months of symptom onset

Clinical Presentation: PD is the second most common neurodegenerative disease (after Alzheimer disease) and is caused by the deposition of alpha-synuclein in the pigmented nuclei of the brainstem. The shelf exam will test your ability to recognize the diagnostic features of Parkinson disease and the available therapies. In addition, PD patients sometimes develop dementia and some patients with Parkinson symptoms develop dementia very early in their disease course. These patients will have more widespread alpha-synuclein deposition and be diagnosed with LBD. Parkinson can also be considered a **hypo**kinetic movement disorder.

The chief complaint will likely be one of four: bradykinesia, resting tremor, postural instability, or cogwheel rigidity. There is a possible link to repeated head trauma and organophosphate exposure may increase risk (toxic to dopaminergic substantia nigra neurons).

PPx: None

MoD: Loss of dopaminergic neurons in the basal ganglia and substantia nigra pars compacta with alpha-synuclein inclusions

Dx:
1. Clinical exam demonstrating tetrad of Parkinson features (see Chapter 17)
2. MRI/CT to r/o mimics of Parkinson disease
   - Normal pressure hydrocephalus may mimic the gait and postural instability of Parkinson disease and can be treated with an LP

Tx/Mgmt:

Treatment cannot reverse the alpha-synuclein pathology, but focuses on symptom management.
   - Levo-carbidopa (carbidopa does not enter the central nervous system (CNS) and blocks degradation of L-dopa outside the CNS)

QUICK TIPS

Parkinson Disease and Huntington Disease are discussed in more detail in Chapter 17

- Dopamine agonists (bromocriptine), less potent than L-dopa
- Deep brain stimulation if L-dopa fails

C. Progressive Supranuclear Palsy (aka Steele-Richardson-Olszewski Syndrome)

Buzz Words: Unable to look down without moving neck + progressive rigidity + dementia + pseudobulbar (lips/tongue/pharyngeal/laryngeal muscles) palsy → progressive supranuclear palsy of oculomotor function

Clinical Presentation: Identifying patients with progressive supranuclear palsy is typically straightforward: look for patients who are unable to move their eyes in the vertical direction in the setting of dementia. The chief complaint may be unsteady gait/imbalance with development of ocular signs (loss of voluntary vertical movements), dystonia of neck muscles, slurred speech, and dysphagia.

PPx: None

MoD: Idiopathic, but neurons in basal ganglia and brainstem are seen to degenerate with phosphorylated tau present.

Dx:

1. Clinical exam to differentiate from Parkinson disease (looking for ocular palsies/dystonia/pseudobulbar signs)
2. MRI may show atrophy of midbrain (in late cases)

Tx/Mgmt:

1. Supportive care
2. Levodopa only slightly effective for rigidity/akinesia
3. Benztropine/botulin injections for dystonia

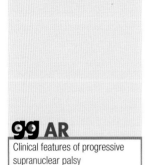

99 AR
Clinical features of progressive supranuclear palsy

D. Huntington Disease

Buzz Words: Atrophy of the caudate nucleus + forgetfulness + family history of early death + change in personality + chorea + depression → HD

Clinical Presentation: HD is the most high-yield disorder of this chapter given how frequently it appears on multiple shelf exams. It is an autosomal dominant condition caused by CAG repeat expansions in the *huntingtin* gene. Patients exhibit wild jerking movements (chorea) and dementia as its prominent features. Many patients develop depression and the suicide rate is quite high. No effective therapies exist. HD can also be considered a **hyper**kinetic movement disorder. The patient's chief complaint may be personality, which emerge first (depression, impulsivity, irritability) and diminished attention/concentration with preserved memory. Patients can also appear "fidgety" with later develop-

99 AR
Choreiform Movements

ment of widespread chorea. There is a family history of chorea/early death. The disease manifests at younger ages with each generation (anticipation, see later for explanation)

PPx:

Genetic testing for counseling

MoD: CAG repeats in the Huntington gene on chromosome 4 expand during replication → increasing lengths = more severe/younger onset of disease → CAG expansion = expansion of polyglutamine region of huntingtin protein → proteins aggregate in neuron nuclei → loss of GABA- and ACh-containing neurons in basal ganglia → atrophy of caudate and putamen

- The mutant huntingtin protein may also interrupt transcriptional proteins or sensitize cells to glutamate excitotoxicity

Dx:

1. Family history with genetic testing for CAG repeats (>39) (2) CT/MRI with atrophy of caudate/putamen and enlarged ventricles

Tx/Mgmt:

Treatment focuses on controlling the chorea

- Haloperidol (dopamine antagonist)
- Tetrabenazine/reserpine (decrease dopamine release as VMAT inhibitors)

Neurodegenerative Disorders Secondary to Systemic Conditions

A. Vascular Dementia

Buzz Words: Sudden, stepwise decrease in memory/cognition + focal neurologic findings

Clinical Presentation: Patients with vascular dementia are older than 40 years and exhibit cognitive decline (dementia) that advances stroke by stroke (stepwise). Risk factors for stroke (high blood pressure, diabetes, atrial fibrillation).

PPx: (1) Stroke prevention (aspirin, statin, anticoagulants for atrial fibrillation [Afib]), (2) risk factors include HTN, Afib, CAD

MoD: (1) Caused by ischemic/hemorrhagic infarcts in multiple brain areas (thalami, basal ganglia, brainstem, cortex)

Dx:

1. MMSE with temporal association between cognitive decline and strokes
2. R/o reversible causes of dementia
3. CT/MRI shows multiple lesions of cortex/subcortical structures

> **QUICK TIPS**
>
> Anticipation = earlier onset in successive generations. During meiosis the CAG repeats can expand so children may have longer expansions than the parents.

Tx/Mgmt:

Treatment focuses on preventing recurrent strokes (see earlier)

B. HIV-Associated Dementia (aka HIV-Associated Neurocognitive Disorder)

Buzz Words: Progressive cognitive problems, including memory loss + immunocompromised young adult + neutropenia + acute onset of symptoms → HIV-associated dementia

Clinical Presentation: On the neurology shelf, patients with HIV (or AIDS-defining illnesses like *Pneumocystis jiroveci* pneumonia) and memory issues should be considered to have HIV-associated dementia until proven otherwise. This is a later stage complication of HIV that presents as subacute progressive dementia with decreased memory and attention, apathy, loss of coordination of limbs, and ataxic gait.

PPx: (1) Treatment of HIV with HAART

MoD: Diffuse rarefaction (decreased density) of cerebral white matter → may be a direct result of infection by HIV

Dx:

1. CD4 count
2. Complete blood count
3. CT/MRI to r/o PML

Tx/Mgmt:

1. HAART

Global Cerebral Dysfunction Disorders

Global cerebral dysfunction disorders are those that tend to affect the cerebrum as a whole (although there are exceptions, such as delirium secondary to hepatic encephalopathy). These disorders are more rarely tested, but appear as distractor answer choices and challenge your knowledge of other diseases. Thus, be familiar with **delirium** and how it differentiates from dementia (dementia is persistent, delirium waxes and wanes) and psychosis (normal electroencephalogram [EEG] vs. abnormal EEG in delirium).

A. Delirium

Buzz Words: Fluctuating mental status (vs. dementia, which is persistent) + sundowning (worse at night) + acute onset + impaired consciousness + visual hallucinations → Delirium

Clinical Presentation: Patients with delirium present with agitation, hallucinations, tremulousness, incoherent thought, and are distracted and disoriented. They frequently have prior alcohol/sedative drug use (looking for delirium in setting of withdrawal).

PPx:
1. Let patient sleep through the night (no 5 a.m. labs)
2. Stop unnecessary meds
3. Decrease stimuli
4. Orient patient to room with calendar and clock

MoD: Caused by many medical insults, including alcohol withdrawal, hypoxemia, intracranial bleeding, infection (both sepsis and primary brain infections), and medications (anticholinergics, benzos)

Dx:
1. Clinical
2. CT/MRI to r/o structural abnormalities
3. EEG (to r/o seizure), but if taken will show diffuse background slowing (vs. psychosis, which has a normal EEG)

Tx/Mgmt:
1. Delirium PPx (e.g., let patient sleep, stop unnecessary meds, decrease stimuli, orient patient with calendar and clock)
2. Haloperidol, quetiapine for acute agitation
3. **Avoid benzos** in the **elderly**, although can be given in young patients

B. Amnestic Disorder

Buzz Words: Isolated amnesia + underlying medical condition + immediately postop + benzos during surgery + cannot learn new information or recall old + confabulation → amnestic disorder

Clinical Presentation: See Buzz Words.

PPx: Avoid precipitating meds like benzos.

MoD: Meds (e.g., Benzos) + trauma + tumor + alcohol + multiple sclerosis

Dx:
1. Medical workup (look for abnormal electrolytes)
2. UDS to look for medications
3. CT/MRI to look for structural lesion

Tx/Mgmt:
None

C. Transient Global Amnesia

Buzz Words: Amnesia + can't learn new info + lasts several hours + **personal identity remains intact**

Clinical Presentation: The key to identifying transient global amnesia is to recognize that personal identity remains intact. On the other hand, dissociative fugue patients lose their personal identification. The chief complaint is normal behavior with amnesia (may manifest as repeti-

tive questioning) and consciousness remains normal.
May be associated with history of migraines.

PPx: Avoid a precipitating insult (such as benzos).

MoD: Unknown, but similar presentation could result
from focal seizure, transient ischemic event, or
migraine.

Dx:
1. Medical workup (look for electrolyte abnormality)
2. UDS to look for medications
3. EEG to rule out seizure
4. CT/MRI to look for structural lesion

Tx/Mgmt:
None, patients usually recover spontaneously

D. Dissociative Amnesia (One Episode)

Buzz Words: One episode of memory or identity loss not
explained by forgetfulness + causes impairment/dis-
tress (patients are aware) + stressful event (patient with
a history of child abuse) → dissociative amnesia

Clinical Presentation: Patients with dissociative amnesia
have a loss of identity with amnesia and are distressed.
There is usually a history of a significant stressor (e.g.,
finding out news of a divorce).

PPx: None

MoD: Unknown

Dx:
1. Rule out other causes of amnesia (epilepsy, concussion, transient global amnesia, acute psychosis).
   • With epilepsy, concussion, and psychosis, the patient will be less responsive/alert.

Tx/Mgmt:
1. Hypnosis to retrieve memory
2. Midazolam (used to reveal memories of what occurred
during amnestic spell)
3. Psychotherapy

E. Dissociative Fugue (Hours to Years)

Buzz Words: Loss of memory and personal identification
(vs. transient global amnesia) + sudden travel from
home + assumes new identity + unaware of illness +
causes marked impairment/distress

Clinical Presentation: Patients with dissociative fugue lose
their personal identity with marked impairment/dis-
tress. There is no history of substance abuse/neurolog-
ic conditions (dissociative fugue is not directly caused
by a substance/other neurologic disorder).

PPx: None

MoD: Unknown

Dx:

1. Medical workup (including UDS)
2. CT/MRI (because head trauma often precedes these cases)

Tx/Mgmt:

1. Hypnosis to retrieve memory
2. Midazolam (used to reveal memories of what occurred during amnestic spell)
3. Psychotherapy

GUNNER PRACTICE

1. A previously healthy 62-year-old man is brought to the physician by his wife because of confusion for 3 hours. During breakfast, he stopped eating and asked his wife the date and plans for the day. He repeated his questions six times despite receiving the correct information from his wife. He now is oriented and thinking clearly. He does not recall any aspect of the morning since breakfast. Physical and mental status examinations show no abnormalities. Which of the following is the most likely diagnosis?
   A. Communicating hydrocephalus
   B. Concussion
   C. Dementia, Alzheimer type
   D. Herpes simplex encephalitis
   E. Hypoxic-ischemic encephalopathy
   F. Hysterical amnesia
   G. Transient global amnesia
   H. Wernicke-Korsakoff syndrome

2. A 61-year-old man presents to the clinic with a several-month history of seeing tiny forest animals in his bedroom, which he describes with amusement. His wife notes that he has not been sleeping well for a while and often kicks and thrashes in bed, sometimes falling out. She also thinks he has been more forgetful and confused. An examination reveals a decreased MMSE with a slight resting tremor and cogwheel rigidity. Which of the following answer choices is correct?
   A. Haloperidol should be prescribed for hallucinations.
   B. An autopsy would likely show alpha-synuclein limited to the substantia nigra.
   C. Levo-carbidopa should be started for resting tremor.
   D. An acetylcholinesterase inhibitor may be used to improve cognitive issues.

3. A 70-year-old woman is seen by her primary care doctor for memory failure and apathy. Her son states that she has been having trouble with her daily activities, including bathing and cleaning her apartment, for the last several months. She frequently forgets her keys and is often unable to keep up with conversations between multiple people. Once an avid gardener, she now rarely tends her plot in the local community garden, saying she is too tired. She previously lived with her husband until his death 5 years prior, and now lives in an assisted living community. She does poorly on the mini-mental exam, but does not appear to put much effort into the questions. When attempting to fold a piece of paper during the exam her hands appear to tremble. Which of the following is the best course of action?
   A. Lumbar puncture to measure the cerebrospinal fluid (CSF) amyloid/tau ratio
   B. Measurement of TSH levels
   C. Urine drug screen
   D. Prescribe Donepezil to improve cognitive decline
   E. Initiate Levo-carbidopa for the tremor

Notes

ANSWERS: What Would Gunner Jess/Jim Do?

1. WWGJD? A previously healthy 62-year-old man is brought to the physician by his wife because of confusion for 3 hours. During breakfast, he stopped eating and asked his wife the date and plans for the day. He repeated his questions six times despite receiving the correct information from his wife. He now is oriented and thinking clearly. He does not recall any aspect of the morning since breakfast. Physical and mental status examinations show no abnormalities. Which of the following is the most likely diagnosis?

Answer: G, Transient global amnesia.

Explanation: This is a classic question stem for transient global amnesia. First, one can rule out chronic or progressive diseases by seeing that the patient's confusion lasted only "for 3 hours." Thus, the only remaining viable answers include concussion, hysterical amnesia, and transient global amnesia. Since there is no history of head trauma, concussion (B) can also be eliminated. Finally, hysterical amnesia is synonymous with pure **retrograde** amnesia, i.e., the patient cannot recall past events. However, patients with hysterical amnesia can remember new information. Thus, the fact that this patient could not learn the "day's date" despite repeating his questions "six times" means it is more likely to be transient global amnesia, in which the patient typically cannot learn anything new.

A. Communicating hydrocephalus → Incorrect. Although hydrocephalus can lead to memory loss (e.g., NPH), it is not transient in symptoms and would show other signs of increased ICP (i.e., Cushing reflex). This patient's "physical and mental status examinations show no abnormalities."

B. Concussion → Incorrect. No history of head trauma rules out this answer choice.

C. Dementia, Alzheimer type → Incorrect. The symptoms only lasted for 3 hours. By definition, dementia is a constant ongoing process. Transient memory loss immediately shifts the differential to global cerebral dysfunction, such as delirium and amnestic disorders.

D. Herpes simplex encephalitis → Incorrect. There are no signs of fever or meningitis as is typically seen in herpes simplex encephalitis patients. Patients with herpes simplex encephalitis certainly would not have normal exams.

E. Hypoxic-ischemic encephalopathy (HIE) → Incorrect. Encephalopathy by definition gives an abnormal mental status exam and does not resolve after a period of only a few hours. HIE is most commonly seen in newborns who do not get enough oxygen to the brain, leading to defects such as cerebral palsy.

F. Hysterical amnesia → Incorrect. As mentioned above, hysterical amnesia patients can learn new information, which this patient cannot.

H. Wernicke-Korsakoff syndrome → Incorrect. Wernicke-Korsakoff syndrome is 2/2 alcohol abuse, which this patient does not have.

2. **WWGJD?** A 61-year-old male presents to the clinic with a several-month history of seeing tiny forest animals in his bedroom, which he describes with amusement. His wife notes that he has not been sleeping well for a while and often kicks and thrashes in bed, sometimes falling out. She also thinks he has been more forgetful and confused. An examination reveals a decreased MMSE with a slight resting tremor and cogwheel rigidity. Which of the following answer choices is correct?

Answer: D, An acetylcholinesterase inhibitor may be used to improve cognitive issues. Explanation: This question tests knowledge of Lewy body dementia. The patient presents with visual hallucinations that do not cause distress and he has been very active during sleep (REM sleep disorder). His wife points out memory problems and confusion, and an exam shows Parkinson signs (resting tremor and cogwheel rigidity). The constellation of dementia with Parkinsonian symptoms, visual hallucinations, and REM sleep behavior is indicative of Lewy body dementia. In this condition, acetylcholinesterase inhibitors (like Donepezil) may be used to try to slow the decline in cognitive function. Acetylcholinesterase inhibitors may also help reduce visual hallucinations.

A. Haloperidol should be prescribed for hallucinations → Incorrect. Older antipsychotics (neuroleptics) should be avoided in patients with Lewy body dementia, because they may cause extreme reactions, such as neuroleptic malignant syndrome or worsening Parkinson symptoms.

B. An autopsy would likely show alpha-synuclein limited to the substantia nigra → Incorrect. In Lewy body dementia, alpha-synuclein inclusions (Lewy bodies) are seen in the substantia nigra, but they are also spread throughout the cortex. In Parkinson disease, alpha synuclein is generally limited to the substantia nigra and other pigmented nuclei of the brainstem.

C. Levo-carbidopa should be started for resting tremor → Incorrect. While levo-carbidopa may be employed to treat Parkinsonian symptoms in Lewy body dementia, it may cause delirium or worsening hallucinations. Because the patient's resting tremor and rigidity are fairly subtle (picked up on exam only), this treatment modality may be delayed until needed.

3. WWGJD? A 70-year-old woman is seen by her primary care doctor for memory failure and apathy. Her son states that she's been having trouble with her daily activities, including bathing and cleaning her apartment, for the last several months. She frequently forgets her keys and is often unable to keep up with conversations between multiple people. Once an avid gardener, she now rarely tends her plot in the local community garden, saying she is too tired. She previously lived with her husband until his death five years prior, and recently moved to an assisted living community. She does poorly on the mini-mental exam, but does not appear to put much effort into the questions. When attempting to fold a piece of paper during the exam her hands appear to tremble. Which of the following is the best course of action?

Answer: B, Measurement of TSH levels

Explanation: This patient is experiencing memory troubles in the context of low energy and apathy after moving to an assisted living community. Although her cognitive issues could be due to Alzheimer disease, her clinical picture should raise concern for depression. She has low energy, exhibits loss of interest in activities she previously found pleasurable, and scores poorly on the MMSE but shows poor effort. Depression could be a product of recent life events (losing a spouse and moving) or could reflect an underlying disorder, such as hypothyroidism. Ordering a TSH along with labs assessing nutritional status would be the best first step of the options presented.

A. Lumbar puncture to measure the CSF amyloid/tau ratio → Incorrect. Alzheimer disease may show a low amyloid/tau ratio in the CSF. This test is not routinely used in the diagnosis of Alzheimer disease and this patient has clues pointing to a reversible cause of dementia, which should be addressed before pursing an invasive test.

C. Urine drug screen → Incorrect. The history provided does not indicate that the patient is taking drugs of abuse.
D. Prescribe Donepezil to improve cognitive decline → Incorrect. This may help if the cognitive decline can be attributed to Alzheimer disease, but there are better explanations for her clinical picture.
E. Initiate Levo-carbidopa for the tremor → Incorrect. Although the patient does have a tremor, it is an action tremor, not a resting tremor. This describes an essential tremor, a common condition in older individuals. Propanolol, not Levo-carbidopa, can be used to treat an essential tremor.

Paroxysmal Disorders

Leo Wang, Hao-Hua Wu, and Chuang-Kuo Wu

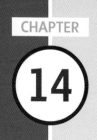

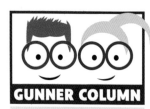

The two main topics of this chapter are headaches and seizures. Both topics are high yield and frequently tested. Headaches, for instance, may also show up on other shelf exams, such as Medicine, Pediatrics, and Family Medicine. When pressed for time, (1) make sure that you can differentiate migraines, tension headaches, and cluster headaches based on buzz words present in the question stem; (2) master temporal arteritis; and (3) know that ethosuximide is the treatment for absence seizures. In addition, please do not memorize all the anti-epileptic drugs; only a few high-yield ones as highlighted in the chapter will be tested.

Headaches

Primary Headaches

Primary headaches are very easy to distinguish. Of the primary headaches, the three most common are migraine, tension, and cluster headaches. These are easily distinguished due to the presence of buzz words. Remember the only bilateral presenting primary headache is the tension headache. The tension headache is also the most common and the only headache that is related to stress. Remember the only one with any sort of genetic predisposition is migraines. Cluster headaches are the only headaches that are more common in men and present unilaterally. Use these to help guide your diagnosis, and remember the prophylaxis (PPx), diagnosis (Dx), and treatment for each of these diseases.

A. Migraine

Buzz Words: Woman with unilateral, pulsating pain + nausea + phonophobia + photophobia lasting 4–72 hours + usually with history of migraines in mother/grandmother → Migraines
- Can be with or without aura (scotoma, teichopsia, numbness, tingling)

Clinical Presentation: On the shelf, the typical patient with migraines is a woman in her late teens, early 20s who experiences sensory auras followed by intense headaches associated with photophobia. This is a high-yield topic so make sure to memorize the diagnostic and management steps as well.

PPx: N/A

MoD: Irritation of CN V, meninges, or blood vessels from vasodilation and due to release of substance P, CGRP, vasoactive peptides from cells in trigeminal nucleus
- Familial migraine caused by deficits in ion channels

Dx:
1. Clinical diagnosis based on two or more repeated headaches for 4–72 hours
2. Computed tomography/magnetic resonance imaging (CT/MRI) only when sudden/severe, after 40, focal neurologic findings to rule out subarachnoid hemorrhage

Tx/Mgmt:
1. Avoid triggers
2. Abortive therapy for few attacks (less than six times per month): triptans (such as sumatriptan), ergotamine
3. Prophylactic treatments for frequent attacks—(if more than six times per month) beta blocker (propranolol), anticonvulsive medicines (i.e., Topiramate)
4. Adjunct therapy: Antidopaminergic drugs (antiemetics/neuroleptics, i.e., metoclopramide, promethazine, and prochlorperazine) for headache and nausea

B. Tension Headache

Buzz Words: Stress-induced + bilateral, band-like pressure around the head

Clinical Presentation: Unlike the other types of headaches, tension headaches are always stress induced on the shelf and presents with a band-like pressure around one's head. There are no accompanying features like nausea, vomiting, photophobia, or phonophobia.

PPx: None

MoD: Unknown, thought to relate to pain filter in brain secondary to stress

Dx:
1. Clinical history

Tx/Mgmt:
1. Nonsteroidal antiinflammatory drugs
2. TCAs
3. Behavioral approaches for stress

C. Cluster Headache

Buzz Words: 1–8 per day + men + extreme irritability and pain + alcohol trigger + autonomic symptoms (lacrimation, pupillary constriction in periorbital and sinus region, unilateral)

Clinical Presentation: Cluster headache is high-yield for the neurology shelf. The classic patient is a young adult male who complains of unilateral headaches that causes his eyes to water. Treatment modalities for cluster headaches are frequently tested.

PPx: N/A

MoD: Dilation of blood vessels → pressure on trigeminal nerve

Dx:

Clinical history and features

Tx/Mgmt:

1. Acute treatments (abortive treatments): 100% oxygen and subcutaneous (SC) Sumatriptan
2. Transitional treatment—steroids
3. Prophylactic treatment—Verapamil, Topiramate, Gabapentin

Secondary Headaches

Secondary headaches are headaches caused by an underlying medical condition. While there are many causes of secondary headaches, most commonly posttraumatic and poststroke-related headaches, the one that is most likely to appear on your shelf is that caused by temporal arteritis. Learn temporal arteritis well and you will get at least one question right on your Neuro, Surgery, and Medicine shelf exams.

A. Temporal Arteritis

Buzz Words: >55 + female + temporal headache + polymyalgia + elevated ESR

Clinical Presentation: Temporal arteritis extremely high-yield because of its multidisciplinary nature (can be seen by specialists ranging from neurologists to rheumatologists to psychiatrists). Any elderly female patient with a temporal headache must be worked up for temporal arteritis, one of the large-vessel vasculitides. Prompt treatment with steroids is essential to preserve eyesight.

PPx: None

MoD: Inflammatory disease of blood vessels → inflames branches of the external carotid artery → occlusion of the ophthalmic artery → irreversible ischemia and blindness if left untreated.

Dx:

1. ESR, CRP, LFTs
2. Biopsy of the temporal artery is diagnostic

Tx/Mgmt:
1. Antiinflammatory steroid not only to treat the pain but prevent blindness

Seizures

Seizure is an important topic. First, recognize that ALL seizures are caused by synchronized neuronal discharge. Second, recognize that many seizures start in the temporal lobe. Some may go on to stay in one area of the brain and are thus called **partial** seizures. Some may go on to recruit neurons of the whole brain and are therefore called **generalized** seizures. Oftentimes, the only way to diagnose the epilepsy syndromes is by electroencephalogram (EEG) recording, but there are certain clinical clues you can use to help you!

Partial Seizure

A. Simple Partial Seizure (Focal Seizure)

Buzz Words: Preserved consciousness + no postictal period + tonic or clonic movement involves only focal portion of body

Clinical Presentation: In simple partial seizures, the consciousness is preserved. Tonic or clonic movements can involve most of the face, neck, or extremities and last 10–20 seconds. There is no postictal period. This entity is not commonly directly tested but will appear as a distractor answer.

PPx: None

MoD: Synchronized neuronal discharge

Dx:
1. EEG shows localized spike and sharp waves

Tx/Mgmt:
1. First line: carbamazepine and valproic acid,
2. Lamotrigine

B. Complex Partial Seizure (Focal Seizure With Consciousness Disturbance)

Buzz Words: Impaired consciousness + postictal period + tonic or clonic movement that involves focal part of body

Clinical Presentation: Complex partial seizures are characterized by tonic or clonic movements involving most of the face, neck, and extremities and lasting 10–20 seconds, accompanied by impaired consciousness.

PPx: None

MoD: Synchronized neuronal discharge

Dx:
1. EEG → Anterior temporal lobe shows sharp waves or focal spikes

Tx/Mgmt:
1. First line: valproic acid, carbamazepine,
2. Lamotrigine

Generalized Seizures

Generalized seizures usually distort activity in the whole or large part of the brain, which is usually characteristic on EEG recording. By definition, generalized seizures impair consciousness. Most begin in childhood and for many patients will go away by adulthood. For those in which it does not go away, they will require lifelong treatment with medications such as valproic acid, lamotrigine, and topiramate. Although there are many new antiepileptic drugs (AEDs) that are considered first line treatment, the shelf exam questions will likely only expect you to know the three mentioned above.

A. Absence Seizure (Petite Mal)

Buzz Words: blank stare + pause in activities for a few seconds + induced by hyperventilation + no memory of event

Clinical Presentation: Guaranteed to be at least one question on your neurology shelf. Patients with absence seizures can present in the question stem as "a kid who does not pay attention" or "zones out easily in class." More common in girls, rare in children < 5 years, rarely lasts longer than 30 seconds. There is no aura or postictal state.

PPx: None

MoD: Dysfunction of T-type calcium channels

Dx:
1. EEG shows 3-per second (3 Hz) typical spike and wave discharges

Tx/Mgmt:
1. Ethosuximide
2. Valproic acid

B. Juvenile Myoclonic Epilepsy (JME)

Buzz Words: Quick, myoclonic jerks of arms + teenager + occurs in morning + followed by clonic-tonic generalized seizure

Clinical Presentation: Only type of seizure that occurs in the morning.

PPx: None

MoD: Synchronized neuronal discharge

Dx:
1. EEG
Tx/Mgmt:
1. Valproic acid

C. Idiopathic Generalized Epilepsy

Buzz Words: Loss of consciousness + skeletal muscles tense, alternating stiffening, and movement + whole body movement

Clinical Presentation: Idiopathic generalized epilepsy is characterized by frequent tonic-clonic seizures (aka grand mal) that involve the whole body. During the episode, the patient's muscles will start to contract and relax rapidly, causing convulsions.

PPx: None
MoD: Synchronized neuronal discharge
Dx:
1. EEG
Tx/Mgmt:
1. Phenytoin
2. Valproic acid

GUNNER PRACTICE

1. A 50-year-old female is brought into the emergency department by her spouse after a generalized tonic-clonic seizure. Patient is unresponsive and examination shows an 8-mm dilated right pupil that is nonreactive to light and drooping of the left lower face. Here, upper and lower extremities of the left side also show decerebrate posturing. Babinski sign is present on the left. What is the most appropriate next step in the management of this patient?
   A. EEG
   B. Antiepileptic medication
   C. CT
   D. MRI
   E. Lumbar puncture
2. A 60-year-old female comes to the physician because her right arm "keeps twitching," sometimes for 3 minutes at a time. Her medical history is significant for stroke, which she was hospitalized for last month. On examination, patient shows mild weakness of her right arm and leg, which has improved since the onset of her stroke. What is the most likely cause of the patient's symptoms?
   A. Psychogenic seizures
   B. Tonic-clonic seizures
   C. Simple partial seizures

D. Conversion disorder

E. Reoccurrence of ischemic stroke

3. A 4-month-old girl is brought into the pediatric emergency department after a 3-minute-long tonic-clonic seizure. Her history is significant for fever and emesis for the past 3 days and difficulty with feeding over the same time period. No other medication besides acetaminophen has been given for the fever. Her blood pressure is 60/40 mm Hg, heart rate is 170/min, and respirations are 40/min. Examination shows a sunken anterior fontanelle and dry mucous membranes. What is the next best diagnostic step?

A. Toxicology screening

B. Measurement of potassium concentration

C. Measurement of calcium concentration

D. Lumbar puncture

E. Culture of blood sample

Notes

ANSWERS: What Would Gunner Jess/Jim Do?

1. WWGJD? A 50-year-old female is brought into the emergency department by her spouse after a **generalized tonic-clonic seizure.** Patient is unresponsive and examination shows a 8-mm dilated right pupil that is nonreactive to light and drooping of the left lower face. Here upper and lower extremities of the left side also show decerebrate posturing. Babinski sign is present on the left. What is the **most appropriate next step** in the management of this patient?

Answer: C, CT

   Explanation: The patient in this question stem most likely has some type of acute intracranial pathology. The first step of a patient with suspected intracranial pathology is to order a CT scan, which can rule out intracranial bleeding. Although the patient was brought into the ED for a seizure, an EEG would not provide any further insight into her acute problem and would not change management. Similarly, while a lumbar puncture can be done to rule out infectious etiologies, typically LPs are performed after neuroimaging. Finally, MRI may be needed to further visualize the vasculature of the brain. However, in acute settings, CT is always the first step.

   A. EEG → Incorrect. Need to rule out life-threatening etiologies first such as intracranial hemorrhage. EEG may be indicated down the line, however.

   B. Antiepileptic medication → Incorrect. While patient may need antiepileptic medications in the future, the cause of her symptoms now may be due to a more emergent condition, such as an intracranial bleed.

   D. MRI → Incorrect. May be done after the CT. In the world of the Neuro shelf, head CT is always done before the head MRI because it is faster and can more rapidly identify emergent etiologies.

   E. Lumbar puncture → Incorrect. Should be performed after neuroimaging if there is suspected subarachnoid hemorrhage.

2. WWGJD? A 60-year-old female comes to the physician because her **right arm "keeps twitching,"** sometimes for 3 minutes at a time. Her medical history is significant for **stroke,** which she was hospitalized for last month. On examination, patient shows mild weakness of her right arm and leg, which has improved since the onset of her

stroke. What is the most likely cause of the patient's symptoms?

Answer: C, simple partial seizures

Explanation: The "twitching" of the arm is likely 2/2 simple partial seizures, which can often occur after a patient has suffered a stroke. Nothing in the history suggested the patient was faking her symptoms, consciously or unconsciously. In addition, it is unlikely a reoccurrence of stroke, since her function, including the weakness, has improved since her discharge from her most recent inpatient stay. Thus, simple partial seizures is the best answer for this question.

A. Psychogenic seizures → Incorrect. Nothing in the question stem suggests the patient is faking her seizures or has any reason to fake her seizures.

B. Tonic-clonic seizures → Incorrect. Patient would not remember her episodes of abnormal movement if she were to have a tonic-clonic seizure.

D. Conversion disorder → Incorrect. Less likely, especially in the setting of a very focal complaint. Typically, patients with conversion disorder complain of more generalized weakness, numbness, or paralysis. Do not be fooled by the patient's "weakness" on exam, which is likely a residual effect of the stroke given that it has improved since last hospitalization.

E. Reoccurrence of ischemic stroke → Incorrect. Less likely, especially given that this patient's symptoms are episodic.

3. WWGJD? A 4-month-old girl is brought into the pediatric emergency department after a 3-minute-long tonic-clonic seizure. Her history is significant for fever and emesis for the past 3 days and difficulty with feeding over the same time period. No other medication besides acetaminophen has been given for the fever. Her blood pressure is 60/40 mmHg, heart rate is 170/min and respirations are 40/min. Examination shows a sunken anterior fontanelle and dry mucous membranes. What is the next best diagnostic step?

Answer: D, lumbar puncture

Explanation: Any patient younger than 6 months with fever needs a lumbar puncture to rule out neurologic infection, such as meningitis. Young patients can often have febrile seizures, but these seizures could also be 2/2 meningitis, which is suspected in this patient. Another common route of infection for a patient this young is through the urinary tract, so a urine culture is typically obtained as well.

A. Toxicology screening → Incorrect. Etiologies for fever, such as meningitis, need to be first ruled out with a lumbar puncture.

B. Measurement of potassium concentration → Incorrect. Etiologies for fever, such as meningitis, need to be first ruled out with a lumbar puncture.

C. Measurement of calcium concentration → Incorrect. Blood test to obtain calcium concentration would take too long to be useful for the initial assessment.

E. Culture of blood sample → Incorrect. Cultures take a very long time and a patient <6 months with fever needs to be worked up for more acute causes.

Sleep Disorders

Hao-Hua Wu, Leo Wang, and Chuang-Kuo Wu

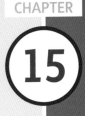

In order to understand sleep disorders, one must learn the normal sleep-wake cycle. There are four stages of sleep:

- Stage 1 (non-REM): Theta waves, muscle tone relaxed, slow eye movements
- Stage 2 (non-REM): K complexes and sleep spindles with no eye movements and little muscle movement
- Stage 3 (non-REM): Delta sleep, low frequency, high voltage, slow wave sleep, deep sleep, most restful sleep, no dream recall
- Stage REM (R): slow, fast voltage on the electroencephalogram (EEG), no muscle tone and rapid eye movements (REM), less restful than stage 3–4, saw tooth waves, vivid dream recall.

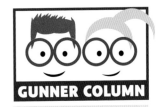

GUNNER COLUMN

Sleep Disorders

Sleep disorders are classified into insomnias (problems with falling asleep), hypersomnias (sleeping too much), or parasomnias (problems during sleep). The most commonly tested sleep disorder is narcolepsy (hypersomnia), which should be the number one take-home point for this chapter. For the other sleep disorders, get a sense of how one differentiates itself from the other, as the Buzz Words are relatively easy to pick. Mechanism of disease and diagnostic steps are less important.

A. Primary Insomnia (≥4 Weeks)

Buzz Words: Fatigue + memory impairment + worries about sleep + sleep interference despite **adequate opportunity to sleep** + impairment of work or daily activity

Clinical Presentation: Patients with primary insomnia cannot fall asleep despite having adequate opportunity to do so, a phenomenon which results in impairment in work and social relationships. Symptoms last for at least four weeks. Management of insomnia is commonly tested so make sure to be familiar with the therapies of choice.

PPx:
1. Good sleep hygiene

MoD: Unknown

Dx:

1. Sleep diary
2. Psych eval (primary insomnia cannot be 2/2 another psych condition)

Tx/Mgmt:

1. Educate about sleep hygiene first, stimulus control therapy, relaxation then CBT
2. Benzos (reduce sleep latency and increase slow wave sleep), such as temazepam
3. Non-benzo hypnotics—Zolpidem, esZopiclone and Zaleplon (three ZZZs for sleeping)
4. Antidepressants such as doxepin
5. Ramelteon (melatonin receptor agonist)

B. Narcolepsy (>3 Months)

Buzz Words: Excessive daytime sleepiness + REM during naps + cataplexy (loss of muscle tone after laughter or extreme emotion) + hallucinations + sleep paralysis when waking up

Clinical Presentation: Narcolepsy is high-yield and extremely likely to show up on your neurology shelf. The Buzz Words that most easily identify this disorder are loss of muscle tone from laughter (cataplexy) or sleep paralysis upon waking up. The treatment of narcolepsy (modafinil, stimulants) is frequently tested.

PPx: Treatment of narcolepsy

MoD: Loss of hypocretin in hypothalamus

Dx:

1. Sleep diary
2. Sleep EEG

Tx/Mgmt:

1. Amphetamine (i.e., dextroamphetamine)
2. Modafinil/Armodafinil
3. Sodium oxybate or desipramine (treatment of cataplexy)
4. Amphetamine-like medicines – Methylphenidate
5. Selective serotonin reuptake inhibitors and TCAs

C. Idiopathic Hypersomnia

Buzz Words: Excessive daytime sleepiness + prolonged nocturnal sleep episodes + frequent urges to nap + occupational and social impairment

Clinical Presentation: Low-yield, but appears frequently as a distractor answer

PPx: None

MoD: Idiopathic

Dx:

1. Sleep diary
2. Sleep EEG

Tx/Mgmt:
1. Improve sleep hygiene
2. Stimulant meds

D. Kleine Levin Syndrome
Buzz Words: Hypersomnia + hyperphagia + hypersexuality + aggression
Clinical Presentation: See Buzz Words.
PPx: None
MoD: Unknown
Dx:
1. Clinical exam
2. Computed tomography/magnetic resonance imaging (CT/MRI) to rule out (r/o) structural lesions
Tx/Mgmt:
1. Stimulants (e.g., modafinil)

E. Circadian Rhythm Sleep Disorders
For these disorders, prophylaxis (PPx) and diagnosis (Dx) are not tested. Instead, know the buzz words, mechanism, and treatment for each circadian rhythm sleep disorder subtype.
MoA:
1. Dysregulation of suprachiasmatic nucleus in the hypothalamus
Buzz Words for Subtypes:
1. Delayed sleep phase disorder (night owl)
   - Delay in sleep onset and awakening times with preserved quality and duration caused by puberty, caffeine, irregular schedules
   - Treat with light therapy, melatonin, and chronotherapy
2. Advanced sleep phase disorder (early sleeper)
   - Normal duration and quality with earlier onset and awakening associated with older age
   - Treat with evening phototherapy
3. Shift-work disorder
   - Misalignment of circadian rhythm from work
   - Tx with bright light therapy to adapt to night shift and modafinil to stay awake
4. Jet lag
   - Sleep disturbance from traveling
   - Self-limiting

F. Sleepwalking (Somnambulism)
Buzz Words: Simple to complex behaviors during slow-wave sleep (deep sleep) + eyes open and glassy look + confusion on awakening with amnesia of event
Clinical Presentation: Patient is confused when waking up from an episode of sleepwalking.

PPx: None

MoD: Unknown

Dx:

1. History from coinhabitant

Tx/Mgmt:

1. Clonazepam (Benzos)
2. TCA

G. Sleep Terrors (Stage 3)

Buzz Words: Episodes of sudden arousal in complete terror with screaming during **slow-wave sleep** + return to sleep w/o awakening + **no memory** of episode

Clinical Presentation: Very frequently tested because it is very similar to nightmare disorder. The key difference is that patients with sleep terrors do not remember their dream whereas those with nightmare disorder do.

PPx: None

MoD: Related to sympathetic hyperactivation and increased muscle tone

Tx/Mgmt:

1. Benzos
2. Protect from injuring themselves during episodes

H. Nightmare Disorder

Buzz Words: Frightening dreams that cause awakening with vivid recall + Related to posttraumatic stress disorder (PTSD) and women

Clinical Presentation: Patients with nightmare disorder **remember** their nightmare (as opposed to patients with sleep terrors).

PPx: Tx of PTSD

MoD: Related to prior trauma

Tx/Mgmt:

1. Imagery rehearsal therapy
2. Antidepressants for severe cases
   • **Not treated with benzos** because this occurs in different stage of sleep

I. REM Behavior Disorder

Buzz Words: Muscle atonia during REM sleep and complex motor activity with dream mentation + sleep talking, yelling, kicking spouse (aka periodic leg movement disorder) + recall of dreams

Clinical Presentation: A very commonly tested disease. The story will always be told by patient's significant other, who gives the most important buzz word of kicking/punching during sleep.

PPx: None
MoD: Can be associated with Parkinson or be idiopathic
Tx/Mgmt:
1. R/o medical conditions (iron anemia, chronic kidney disease, neuropathy)
2. Clonazepam (first line of treatment)
3. Dopamine agonists (i.e., pramipexole, ropinirole)
4. Carbamazepine
5. Levodopa

J. Restless Legs Syndrome

Buzz Words: Irresistible urge to move legs + urge is relieved when patient moves legs + impairs sleep + leads to nocturnal awakenings

Clinical Presentation: Restless legs syndrome (RLS) is considered a movement disorder instead of a sleep disorder. However, it can cause one to present like a sleep disorder (e.g., nonrestful sleep) due to an irresistible urge to move the legs. Thus, it is important to have RLS in your differential for sleep disorders. Periodic limb movements in sleep (PLMS) or periodic limb movement disorder (PLMD), on the other hand, is characterized by patients with repetitive 30-second twitching of legs or arms during sleep and is associated with REM behavior disorder.

PPx: None
MoD: Unknown but may be related to dopamine dysfunction
Dx:
1. History from patient and coinhabitant
2. Polysomnography to r/o PLMD
Tx/Mgmt:
1. Pramipexole, ropinirole
2. Rotigotine patch
3. Gabapentin
4. Iron supplements if Fe anemia

GUNNER PRACTICE

1. A 47-year-old woman comes to the physician because of daily "crawling tightness" in her calves for 5 years. She notices the discomfort when she sits up for long periods of time or lies in bed. The discomfort prevents her from falling asleep quickly. She reports that if she stands and walks, she obtains temporary relief. She is otherwise healthy and takes no medications. Peripheral pulses are normal. Neurologic examination shows no abnormalities. Which of the following is the most appropriate pharmacotherapy?
   A. Carbamazepine
   B. Clopidogrel

C. Naproxen

D. Pramipexole

E. Quinine

F. No pharmacotherapy indicated

2. A 32-year-old man comes to his primary care physician complaining of a 4-month history losing consciousness every time he laughs. He sleeps 10 hours every evening and gets vivid nightmares. During the day, he is tired and drowsy. Recently, he was involved in a motor vehicle collision from which he suffered no injuries. Physical exam is unremarkable. Which of the following is the most likely diagnosis?

A. Absence seizure

B. Complex partial seizure

C. Malingering

D. Narcolepsy

E. Sleep apnea

F. Sleep terror disorder

G. Major depressive disorder (MDD)

3. A 43-year-old man comes to the physician because of drowsiness during the day. His wife says he sometimes gets up in the middle of the evening and leaves the bedroom. He has no recollection of these episodes in the morning. There are no abnormal findings during his sleep study. What is the most appropriate next step in management?

A. Clonazepam

B. Clonidine

C. Carbamazepine

D. Bromocriptine

E. Pramipexole

Notes

ANSWERS: What Would Gunner Jess/Jim Do?

1. WWGJD? A 47-year-old woman comes to the physician because of daily "crawling tightness" in her calves for 5 years. She notices the discomfort when she sits up for long periods of time or lies in bed. The discomfort prevents her from falling asleep quickly. She reports that if she stands and walks, she obtains temporary relief. She is otherwise healthy and takes no medications. Peripheral pulses are normal. Neurologic examination shows no abnormalities. Which of the following is the most appropriate pharmacotherapy?

Answer: D, Pramipexole

Explanation: This patient is suffering from **RLS**, which can be ascertained by her "crawling tightness" in her calves that is only relieved when she "stands and walks" but prevents her from "falling asleep quickly." Although the mechanism is unclear, RLS is thought to be 2/2 dopamine dysfunction. Thus, it is treated with dopamine agonists, such as pramipexole (D).

A. Carbamazepine → Incorrect. Carbamazepine is an antiepileptic drug most commonly used for treatment of trigeminal neuralgia.

B. Clopidogrel → Incorrect. Clopidogrel is an antiplatelet agent used to prevent thrombosis or stroke.

C. Naproxen → Incorrect. Naproxen is a long-acting nonsteroidal antiinflammatory drug used to treat pain.

E. Quinine → Incorrect. Quinine is an antimalarial drug derived from tree bark.

F. No pharmacotherapy indicated → Incorrect. Pharmacotherapy is indicated in RLS.

2. WWGJD? A 32-year-old man comes to his primary care physician complaining of a 4-month history losing consciousness every time he laughs. He sleeps 10 hours every evening and gets vivid nightmares. During the day, he is tired and drowsy. Recently, he was involved in a motor vehicle collision from which he suffered no injuries. Physical exam is unremarkable. Which of the following is the most likely diagnosis?

Answer: D. Narcolepsy

Explanation: Losing consciousness during laughing is almost pathognomonic for narcolepsy. Hallucinations and daytime sleepiness are also common. The mechanism for this is loss of hypocretin in the hypothalamus.

The drowsiness in this man most likely contributed to his motor vehicle collision.

A. Absence seizure → Incorrect. There is no evidence to suggest a seizure disorder. Absence seizures are not precipitated by laughing.

B. Complex partial seizure → Incorrect. There is no evidence to suggest a seizure disorder.

C. Malingering → Incorrect. Malingering is a possibility but there is no secondary gain and the presentation fits that of narcolepsy much better.

D. Sleep apnea → Incorrect. Sleep apnea would cause daytime drowsiness, but does not explain a loss of consciousness from laughter.

F. Sleep terror disorder → Incorrect. Vivid nightmares can be explained by sleep terror disorder but does not explain his loss of consciousness every time he laughs and his drowsiness during the day.

G. MDD → Incorrect. There is no evidence for MDD in this patient besides daytime drowsiness and excessive sleeping.

3. WWGJD? A 43-year-old man comes to the physician because of drowsiness during the day. His wife says he sometimes gets up in the middle of the evening and leaves the bedroom. He has no recollection of these episodes in the morning. There are no abnormal findings during his sleep study. What is the most appropriate next step in management?

Answer: A. Clonazepam

Explanation: This man is losing sleep because he is sleepwalking during the night, also known as somnambulism. The treatment for sleepwalking is clonazepam, followed by a TCA if needed. Most sleepwalkers are brought in by a family member.

B. Clonidine → Incorrect, not indicated for sleep walking. Clonidine is used for ADHD and anxiety.

C. Carbamazepine → Incorrect, not indicated. This antiepileptic is used for bipolar disorder and neuropathic pains.

D. Bromocriptine → Incorrect, not indicated. Bromocriptine is used for a number of dopamine related disorders, especially in the pituitary.

E. Pramipexole → Incorrect, not indicated. Pramipexole is used for RLS.

Notes

Neuromuscular Disorders

Michael Baer, Leo Wang, Hao-Hua Wu,
and Chuang-Kuo Wu

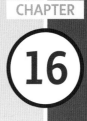

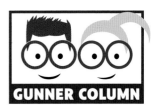

GUNNER COLUMN

Neuromuscular disorders are frequently tested on the neurology shelf exam. These disorders can seem confusing if they are approached without a strong organizational framework. Like most of neurology, the initial step when evaluating a patient is to localize the problem to a specific anatomical level. Neuromuscular disorders are especially geared to this approach. When studying these diseases and answering questions try to look for: (1) presence of **upper** or **lower** motor neuron disease, (2) signs of neuromuscular junction damage, or (3) clues of a myopathy. This will allow you to quickly narrow a differential from the large list of possibilities. The **pattern** of weakness is also important to consider, as many of these diseases have pathognomonic distributions of involvement. Lastly, neuromuscular disorders require a firm grasp on disease mechanism, as this guides diagnosis and treatment. For example, myasthenia gravis is caused by the reversible blockage of acetylcholine receptors with antibodies; therefore, one diagnostic step involves measuring levels of antibodies against the postsynaptic acetylcholine receptor, and treatment involves increasing synaptic acetylcholine to overcome the reversible blockage.

Diseases of Upper and Lower Motor Neurons

A. Amyotrophic Lateral Sclerosis (ALS, Lou Gehrig Disease)

Buzz Words: Worsening weakness (distal > proximal) + stiffness + muscle wasting and fasciculations + hyperreflexia + eventual difficulty speaking, swallowing, breathing

Clinical Presentation: ALS is an incredibly debilitating disease with no curative treatment. Look for an elderly person presenting with weakness and signs of both upper and lower motor neuron damage (Table 16.1). Postmortem examination will reveal loss of the nerve cells in the anterior horns of the spinal cord, the motor nuclei of the brainstem, and the motor cortex. Ten percent of cases are familial and several causative

TABLE 16.1 Upper Motor Neuron Versus Lower Motor Neuron Symptoms and Signs

	Lower motor neuron	Upper motor neuron
Deep tendon reflexes	Absent	Increased
Pathologic reflex	Absent	Present
Atrophy	Present	Less prominent early
Fasciculations	Present	Absent

TABLE 16.2 Key Electromyography Findings/Terms

Term	Definition
Motor unit	Lower motor neuron and all the muscle fibers it innervates
Motor unit potential (MUP)	Electrical signal generated by one motor unit
Myopathic pattern	Decreased MUP due to death of muscle fibers
Denervation	Damage of motor neuron axon leads to loss of innervation of its muscle fibers
Reinnervation	Undamaged axons sprout connections to denervated muscle fibers (creates bigger motor units)
Giant polyphasic potential	Large MUP due to larger motor units from reinnervation

mutations have been identified. Riluzole is the only agent that gives a short gain in survival.

PPx: None

MoD: Due to loss of the motor neurons in the anterior horn of the spinal cord, brainstem motor nuclei, and motor cortex. Inclusions of the TDP-43 protein (RNA binding protein, also in FTLD) are seen in most cases.

- Familial cases (mainly autosomal dominant) caused by repeat expansions of *C9orf72* gene, mutations in *SOD1* (superoxide dismutase 1) and *TARDBP* (TDP-43).

Dx:

1. Exam with triad of weakness and atrophy of affected limb, fasciculations + spasticity of limb, generalized hyperreflexia
2. Electromyography (EMG) with enlarged motor units (indicates reinnervation) and fibrillations (active denervation) (Table 16.2)
3. Computed tomography/magnetic resonance imaging (CT/MRI) (if concerned about structural spinal problem, i.e., ruptured cervical disc)
4. Muscle biopsy (not always necessary, will show neurogenic denervation)

gg AR
Fasciculations in ALS

5. LP
6. Genetic testing for familial types of ALS

Tx/Mgmt:
1. Physical therapy to maintain mobility
2. BiPAP for respiratory failure
3. Riluzole (antiglutamate agent thought to block Na channels in damaged neurons)

Diseases of the Lower Motor Neurons

A. Spinal Muscular Atrophy (Werdnig-Hoffman Disease)

Buzz Words: Weak and limp baby + absent tendon reflexes + poor suck and swallow + family history + worsening respiratory function + death in first year

Clinical Presentation: Spinal muscular atrophy (SMA) is an inherited disease that leads to degeneration of the lower motor neurons and is the second leading cause of death from an autosomal recessive disease (after cystic fibrosis). The most severe form (SMA I) presents at birth or the first few months of life as generalized weakness and hypotonia ("floppy baby"). Death usually occurs in the first year.

PPX: None

MoD: Mutations/deletion of *SMN* gene lead to decreased survival of motor neurons in spinal cord/brainstem motor nuclei

Dx:
1. Genetic sequencing
2. Muscle biopsy demonstrating group atrophy (sign of denervation)
3. EMG with fibrillations

Tx/Mgmt: Supportive care, no curative therapy

Diseases of the Neuromuscular Junction

Two conditions affecting the neuromuscular junction are presented here: myasthenia gravis and Lambert-Eaton myasthenic syndrome (LEMS; Table 16.3). These two conditions are often tested against one another, but careful attention to the clinical presentation helps differentiate the two. Other commonly tested neuromuscular conditions include botulism and tetanus, which are discussed in Chapter 6.

A. Myasthenia Gravis

Buzz Words: Weakness of facial muscles + diplopia + worse with repeated activity, better with rest + ptosis with sustained upgaze + thymoma + acetylcholine receptor antibodies

TABLE 16.3 Myasthenia Gravis Versus Lambert-Eaton Myasthenic Syndrome

	Myasthenia gravis	Lambert-Eaton myasthenic syndrome
Pattern of weakness	Muscles of face	Trunk/lower extremities
Effect of activity	Activity worsens weakness	Activity improves weakness
Associations	Thymoma	Small cell lung cancer
Mechanism	Antibodies against acetyl-choline receptor	Antibodies against presynaptic calcium channel
Therapy	Acetylcholines-terase inhibitors	3,4-Diaminopyridine

QUICK TIPS

Myasthenic crisis = Rapid and severe deterioration of strength, leading to respiratory failure and paralysis. Requires prompt treatment plasma exchange/IVIg!

Clinical Presentation: The predominant feature of myasthenia gravis is fluctuating weakness of the skeletal muscles, notably those of the face, throat, and neck. The key clinical features are weakness with repeated activity, gain in strength with rest, and improved strength with anticholinesterase drugs. A portion of myasthenia gravis patients will also have a thymic tumor.

The most common chief complaint is specific muscular weakness, worsening with repeated use or as the day wears on (i.e., complaints of ptosis, or difficulty fixing hair due to fatigued shoulders).

May see family history of connective tissue diseases (autoimmune).

PPX: None

MoD: Autoantibodies generated to the acetylcholine receptor (on postsynaptic side of NMJ) → binding of autoantibodies blocks action of acetylcholine → antibody bindings leads to degradation of acetylcholine receptors → decreased bindings sites + decreased number of receptors = lower amplitude of postsynaptic potentials at NMJ
  • With repeated use the amount of acetylcholine within the synaptic cleft decreases (less acetylcholine is released with each impulse) → leads to weakness
  • 10% of patients will have thymic tumors and many respond well to thymectomy → thymus may play role in autoimmunity

Dx:
1. Exam with weakness of facial muscles after sustained activity (ptosis with sustained upgaze)
2. Regained strength after period of rest
3. Increased strength with acetylcholinesterase inhibitors (neostigmine and ephodrium)

gg AR
Neuromuscular junction in MG

4. + serum anti-acetylcholine receptor antibodies (80%–90%)
5. EMG showing reduced amplitude of muscle action potentials with repetitive stimulation
6. CT of chest for thymoma

Tx/Mgmt:

1. Acetylcholinesterase inhibitors (neostigmine and pyridostigmine)
2. Immune modulating agents (corticosteroids, azathio-prine)
3. Plasma exchange (severe myasthenia refractory to acetylcholinesterase inhibitors/steroids)
4. IVIg (short term control of worsening myasthenia)
5. Thymectomy (30% remission rate, perform in all patients with thymoma)
   • For myasthenic crisis, secure airway, ventilate, and initiate plasma exchange/IVIg. Anticholinesterase inhibitors and steroids started with weaning from ventilator.

B. Lambert-Eaton Myasthenic Syndrome

Buzz Words: Weakness of trunk/lower extremities + increased power after several contractions + small cell lung cancer

Clinical Presentation: While LEMS also leads to weakness, the pattern is distinctive from myasthenia gravis. LEMS presents with weakness of the muscles of the trunk and lower extremities (difficulty climbing stairs/walking) vs. muscles of the face. With LEMS, there is an **increase** in muscle power after the initial couple contractions, while myasthenia shows a **decrease** in power after initial contractions. LEMS is associated with carcinomas, notably small cell lung cancer, and its diagnosis should prompt a search for a tumor. A common chief complaint is weakness (difficulty rising from chair, climbing up stairs). May have history of tumor, but weakness is often the first sign.

PPx: None

MoD: Autoantibodies generated against the presynaptic voltage-gated calcium channels → Binding of antibodies renders calcium channels nonfunctional → Decreased influx of calcium with nerve impulse → Decreased number of synaptic vesicles fusing with plasma membrane → Decreased acetylcholine in synaptic cleft → Decrease in muscle contractility

Dx:

1. Exam with symmetrical weakness of proximal muscles (legs/hips/shoulders)

QUICK TIPS

Acetylcholinesterase inhibitors MoA = decrease destruction of acetylcholine in synaptic left → more acetylcholine = stronger postsynaptic amplitude and better contraction

QUICK TIPS

Neostigmine = Prostigmin, pyridostigmine = Mestinon

QUICK TIPS

Increased power after first several contractions due to increased calcium in the presynaptic nerve → more acetylcholine release

99 AR

Mechanism of LEMS

2. Increase in strength after first several contractions
3. EMG with increased amplitude of muscle action potentials following voluntary contraction
4. Antibodies against voltage gated calcium channels
5. Screening for malignancy (chest CT to start to r/o small cell lung cancer)

Tx/Mgmt:
1. 3,4-diaminopyridine (3,4-DAP)
2. Immunosuppressive therapy (corticosteroids, azathioprine)
3. Plasmapheresis/IVIg
4. Treat underlying malignancy

Diseases of the Muscle

This is a broad category of diseases in which the primary pathology is localized to the muscle. Disease can occur secondary to inflammation/immunity (inflammatory myopathies), inherited defects leading to degeneration of the muscle (muscular dystrophies), drugs (statin-induced myopathy), and defects in ion channels (muscle channelopathies). Clues that localize a disease to the muscle include muscle weakness, pain and cramping, stiffness, and changes in muscle bulk. Once again, the **pattern** of weakness will be very important (i.e., proximal weakness in Duchenne/Becker muscular dystrophies). An understanding of the diagnostic processes requires a knowledge of the underlying anatomy, so it is worthwhile to review Table 16.2 and the basics of the motor unit.

Inflammatory Myopathies

A. Polymyositis

Buzz Words: Progressive painless proximal weakness (can't get out of chair/combing hair) + connective tissue disease + elevated CK + biopsy with inflammation in endomysium and necrosis

Clinical Presentation: Polymyositis and dermatomyositis are very similar conditions, as either may be associated with a connective tissue disease or an underlying malignancy. Dermatomyositis, however, is set apart by its distinctive heliotrope rash. Patients have a chief complaint of weakness of proximal muscles (can't comb hair/put items on high shelf/rise out of chair). Associated with autoimmune disease (RA/scleroderma/lupus), history of carcinoma (lung/colon in men, breast/ovary in women).

PPx: None

MoD: Idiopathic, but thought to be autoimmune (association with systemic autoimmune conditions and specific autoantibodies)

Dx:

1. Exam with weakness of the proximal muscles
2. Elevated CK
3. Autoantibody titers for systemic autoimmune conditions
4. EMG with "myopathic pattern,"
5. Muscle biopsy with CD8+ T cells in endomysium and myonecrosis

Tx/Mgmt:

1. Corticosteroids (monitor response with CK improvement/motor exam)
2. IVIg and methylprednisolone for severe, acute cases

B. Dermatomyositis

Buzz Words: Proximal muscle weakness + scaly patches over extensor surfaces of joints + papules over DIP and PIP joints (Gottron papules [Fig. 16.1]) + heliotrope rash on face (Fig. 16.2) + shawl sign + biopsy with perimysial B cells

Clinical Presentation: Most common chief complaint is proximal weakness and rash. Associated with autoimmune diseases and carcinomas.

PPx: None

MoD: Idiopathic, but thought to be autoimmune (association with systemic autoimmune conditions and specific autoantibodies)

Dx:

1. Exam with weakness of the proximal muscles and characteristic rash
2. Elevated CK
3. Autoantibody titers for systemic autoimmune conditions
4. EMG with "myopathic pattern,"
5. Muscle biopsy with perimysial B cells and perifascicular atrophy

Tx/Mgmt:

1. Corticosteroids (monitor response with CK improvement/motor exam)
2. IVIg and methylprednisolone for severe, acute cases

C. Inclusion Body Myositis

Buzz Words: Progressive painless proximal and distal weakness + slightly elevated CK + muscle biopsy with CD8+ T cells and vacuoles with basophilic granules (inclusion bodies) + poor response to steroids

QUICK TIPS

Anti-Jo1 + in 20% of PM and DM cases

QUICK TIPS

Endomysium = around individual myofibers, Perimysium = around fiber bundles/fascicles

QUICK TIPS

Shawl sign = rash over shoulders and upper arms

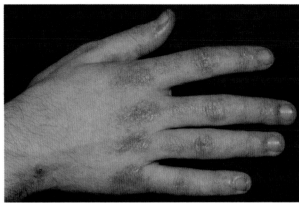

FIG. 16.1 Gottron papules. (Courtesy of Julie V Schaffer, MD. From Jorizzo JL, Vleugels RA. Dermatomyositis. In: Bolognia JL, Jorizzo JL, Schaffer JV, eds. *Dermatology*. 3rd ed. London: Elsevier Ltd; 2012.)

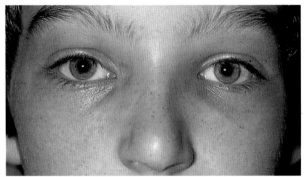

FIG. 16.2 Heliotrope rash. (From Lissauer T, Clayden G, Craft A. Neurological disorders. In: Lissauer T, ed. *Illustrated Textbook of Pediatrics*. 4th ed. London: Elsevier Ltd; 2012.)

Clinical Presentation: Inclusion body myositis (IBM) is the most common inflammatory myopathy over the age of 50. Unlike PM and DM, IBM is not associated with malignancies or systemic autoimmune conditions. A likely chief complaint is proximal/distal weakness of legs, distal weakness of arms (i.e., weakness of wrist flexors). It is associated with diabetes.

PPx: None

MoD: Idiopathic

Dx:

1. Exam with proximal/distal weakness of legs, distal weakness of arms
2. Slightly elevated CK
3. EMG with "myopathic pattern,"
4. Muscle biopsy with CD8+ T cells, vacuole with basophilic granules highlighted by Gomori trichrome stain (inclusion bodies)

Tx/Mgmt: IBM does not respond well to steroids or other immunosuppressives, and IVIg is of limited benefit. With no effective therapies, the disease is generally progressive.

Muscular Dystrophies

The muscular dystrophies refer to a group of hereditary diseases characterized by degeneration of the skeletal muscle. Since covering all the muscular dystrophies would take an entire textbook, only three of the more common diseases are presented here, as they are sure to appear on the shelf exam as well as Step 1 and Step 2.

A. Duchenne Muscular Dystrophy

Buzz Words: Male toddler + foot drop, toe walk, waddling gait + Gowers sign + pseudohypertrophy + severely elevated CK + *dystrophin* mutation + progressive respiratory failure

Gowers' sign

Clinical Presentation: Duchenne muscular dystrophy, inherited with an X-linked recessive pattern, is the most common muscular dystrophy, affecting 1 in 3300 live male births. Weakness begins in early childhood and runs a progressive course, with death occurring in young adulthood. Becker muscular dystrophy is a related but less severe condition, as both are due to mutations in the *dystrophin* gene. Patients present with difficulty walking with waddling, foot drop, toe walking (proximal weakness first).

PPx: None

MoD: Dystrophin protein involved in stabilizing the sarcolemma. Loss of dystrophin leads to damage of sarcolemma → influx of calcium into muscle cells → protease activation and muscle damage

Dx:
1. Exam with proximal weakness and pseudohypertrophy
2. + family history
3. Elevated CK
4. Muscle biopsy with myonecrosis and inflammation (late stages show replacement with fat)
5. Genetic testing for *dystrophin* mutations

Tx/Mgmt: No effective therapies exist. Corticosteroids may give short improvement of muscle strength. Treatment focuses on maintaining strength and respiratory function.

B. Becker Muscular Dystrophy

Buzz Words: Young adult male + progressive proximal weakness + family history of adult onset weakness + elevated CK

QUICK TIPS
Pseudohypertrophy = muscular enlargement due to fatty replacement

QUICK TIPS
Hatchet face = narrowed face due to atrophy of masseters

Clinical Presentation: Becker muscular dystrophy presents with weakness in the same muscles as Duchenne but at a later age and in a less debilitating manner. The condition is due to mutilations in *dystrophin* that lead to an abnormal protein (vs. loss of protein in Duchenne). Like Duchenne patients with BMD present with difficulty walking (waddling, foot drop, toe walking). Proximal weakness comes first.

PPx: None

MoD: Similar to Duchenne muscular dystrophy, but dystrophin is still produced (but abnormally) in Becker.

Dx:
1. Exam with proximal weakness and pseudohypertrophy
2. + family history
3. Elevated CK
4. Muscle biopsy with myonecrosis and inflammation (milder than Duchenne)
5. Genetic testing for *dystrophin* mutations
6. Screening for dilated cardiomyopathy (dystrophin cause dilated cardiomyopathy

Tx/Mgmt: No definitive therapy exists

C. Myotonic Dystrophy

Buzz Words: Atrophy and weakness of small muscles of hand + "hatchet" face + frontal baldness + bradycardia + myotonia + CTG repeat expansion in *DMPK*

Clinical Presentation: Type 1 myotonic dystrophy is the most common adult muscular dystrophy, inherited as an autosomal dominant secondary to trinucleotide repeat expansions in the *DMPK* gene. These patients experience weakness and myotonia (delayed relaxation after strong contraction). The likely chief complaint is atrophy and weakness of small muscles of hand and myotonia. There is likely a family history of myotonic dystrophy with earlier age of onset in each new generation (anticipation).

PPx: None

MoD: CTG repeat expansion of *DMPK* gene → accumulation of enlarged RNA sequences in nucleus → mRNA alternative splicing disrupted → changes in expression of many genes

Dx:
1. Genetic sequencing of CTG repeat length
2. Screening for cardiac conduction abnormalities (bradycardia and P-R block)

Tx/Mgmt: No effective therapy to reverse progression. Pacemaker used for bradycardia or heart block.

Drug Associated Myopathies

A. Statin-Induced Myopathy

Buzz Words: Muscle aches/fatigue + elevated CK + statin use

Clinical Presentation: See Buzz Words

PPx: None

MoD: Unknown, but may be due to a genetic susceptibility rendering certain individuals more likely to experience toxicity from statins

Dx:

1. Concordant clinical history/exam with mildly elevated CK
2. Improvement with discontinuation of statin

Tx/Mgmt: Discontinue the statin and use an alternative agent to lower cholesterol

Muscle Channelopathies

The diseases in this category are due to changes in the movement of ions across the muscle membrane. Two conditions lead to period paralysis, while the other (malignancy hyperthermia) causes an adverse reaction to certain classes of general anesthetics.

A. Hyperkalemic Periodic Paralysis

Buzz Words: Generalized weakness + episodic (after exercise) + in setting of high K + mutation in alpha subunit of Na channel

Clinical Presentation: Both hyperkalemic periodic paralysis and hypokalemic period paralysis can, as their names suggest, cause period paralysis in the setting of different electrolyte abnormalities. The two are easy to distinguish once the underlying pathology is memorized. Patients present with attacks of weakness when resting after exercise.

PPx: Lower serum K levels with (1) acetazolamide or (2) hydrochlorothiazide

MoD: Mutations in Na channel block inactivation → decreased inactivation of Na channel leads to incomplete repolarization → muscle cell is more excitable → with increased depolarizations muscle cell unexcitable → state of paralysis

- Increased K makes the problem worse, because K must leave the muscle cell for repolarization (more K outside the cell, the less K wants to move out the cell)

99 AR

Action potential generation in skeletal muscle

Dx:
1. + provocative test (oral K leads to weakness)
2. Genetic testing for Na channel mutation

Tx/Mgmt:
1. Lower serum K levels to prevent attack
2. IV calcium gluconate for acute attacks (or IV glucose/insulin/hydrochlorothiazide)

B. Hypokalemic Periodic Paralysis

Buzz Words: Attacks of weakness during night/early morning + limbs > trunk + low serum K + mutation in alpha subunit of Ca channel

Clinical Presentation: Patients present with episodes of weakness, generally during early morning hours. They are likely to have a positive family history due to the autosomal dominant inheritance pattern.

PPx:
1. Low Na diet
2. acetazolamide (due to acidosis)
3. K sparing diuretics
4. daily oral K

MoD: Mutation in Ca channel disrupt voltage sensor → more difficult for depolarizations to induce release of Ca from sarcoplasmic reticulum → weakness
- Low serum K precipitates attacks because the muscle cell will repolarize more quickly (lower K outside the cell = greater movement of K from inside to outside cell). Quicker repolarization gives broken Ca channel less time to respond to voltage signal.

Dx:
1. + provocative test (oral glucose/NaCl + exercise = weakness)
2. Genetic testing for Ca channel mutation

Tx/Mgmt:
1. Raise serum K to prevent attack
2. Oral K for acute attack

C. Malignant Hyperthermia

Buzz Words: General anesthesia (halothane) or muscle relaxant (succinylcholine) + rigidity + rising body temp + acidosis + myoglobinuria + elevated CK + high mortality rate + inherited susceptibility

Clinical Presentation: High-yield, also frequently seen on the psychiatry shelf. Patients present with rigidity and increased temperature after inhaled anesthetic or muscle relaxant given

PPx: Avoid halothane or succinylcholine in susceptible individuals (use propofol, barbiturates, or nitrous oxide instead)

MoD: Mutations in ryanodine receptor → increased sensitivity of receptor to halothane → release of calcium from sarcoplasmic reticulum → increased intracellular calcium causes contraction and rigidity

Dx:

1. Close monitoring of patient/vitals after induction with anesthesia
2. Identification of susceptible individuals with family/personal history

Tx/Mgmt:

1. Dantrolene (inhibits Ca release from sarcoplasmic reticulum)
2. Body cooling, IV hydration, NaBicarb (decreases acidosis)

Demyelinating Disorders Mimicking Movement Disorders

A. Multiple Sclerosis (MS)

Buzz Words: Neurologic dysfunction separated in time and space (optic neuritis and internuclear ophthalmoplegia, sensory loss, bladder dysfunction, trigeminal neuralgia, intention tremor) + young woman + Lhermitte sign

Clinical Presentation: MS is a demyelinating disease in which the central nervous system (CNS) is demyelinated. It is named for the *multiple sclerosing plaques* of the white matter in the CNS. The symptoms can be relatively nonspecific, although most patients present with symptoms in the eye. It is unlikely you will be tested on the pathophysiology of MS on the shelf, since this is not well understood. More likely, you will be tested on recognizing, diagnosing, and managing the disease. In this context, having an understanding of the breadth of knowledge of MS is important, especially the different clinical presentations that can affect how the disease presents over long periods of time.

PPx: None

MoD: Thought to be a contribution of environmental and genetic factors related to early childhood virus infection → autoimmune destruction of oligodendrocytes, demyelination occurs in CNS only, thought to related to vitamin D and T cells reactive to myelin basic protein

Dx:

1. Clinical/neurologic exam based on pattern of presentation
2. MRI: white matter lesions that separate in space and time (i.e., a lesion has to appear in two different places at two different times)
3. LP: cerebrospinal fluid (CSF) with oligoclonal bands

Tx/Mgmt:

1. Acute: steroids and plasmapheresis
2. Disease modifying: injectable medicines—IFN-1alpha, IFN-1beta, glatiramer (mimics myelin), natalizumab, ivoral medicines—fingolimod, teriflunomide, dimethyl fumarate
3. Physical therapy

GUNNER PRACTICE

1. A 45-year-old female presents to clinic for fatigue and muscle weakness. She reports difficulty completing her 10-hour workday, because it is difficult to keep her eyelids open. In addition, she has noticed that her ability to grip her coffee mug or carry things around the office is worse in the afternoon. On examination, patient has drooping eyelids at baseline and has weakened strength with repetitive motion. What is the most likely diagnosis?

   A. Lambert Eaton
   B. Myasthenia gravis
   C. Narcolepsy
   D. Multiple sclerosis
   E. Parkinson disease

2. A 60-year-old man comes to the physician with muscle weakness and cramping that has been ongoing for the past 4 months. On exam, the patient was found to have hyperactive deep tendon reflexes, fasciculations, and muscle atrophy in the left and right leg as well as right wrist drop. There were no abnormalities in the sensory or proprioceptive examinations. Given his clinical presentation, what diagnosis does the patient most likely have?

   A. Guillain-Barre syndrome
   B. Cauda equina
   C. Multiple sclerosis
   D. Amyotrophic lateral sclerosis
   E. Myasthenia gravis

3. A 55-year-old female presents to a dermatologist with a violet rash around her eyes and red papules over the joints of her fingers. She notes that she's been feeling tired lately and has been having trouble stocking the

highest shelves while volunteering at the food pantry. She thinks she has lost weight recently and hasn't seen her primary care doctor for several years. When the appointment is over the dermatologist has to help her out of her chair. Which of the following answer choices is correct?

A. Corticosteroids would not be expected to improve the weakness
B. A mammography should be ordered
C. Neostigmine would lead to increased strength
D. A muscle biopsy would show CD8+ T cells in the endomysium

ANSWERS: What Would Gunner Jess/Jim Do?

1. WWGJD? A 45-year-old female presents to clinic for **fatigue and muscle weakness**. She reports difficulty completing her 10-hour workday because it is so difficult to keep her eyelids open. She gets 8 hours of sleep every night and feels well-rested in the morning. In addition, she has noticed that her ability to grip her coffee mug or carry things around the office is **worse in the afternoon**. On examination, patient has **drooping eyelids on baseline and has weakened strength with repetitive motion**. What is the **most likely diagnosis?**

Answer: B, Myasthenia gravis

Explanation: This is a classic question that will test your ability to differentiate myasthenia gravis from Lambert Eaton. In the former, strength of movement diminishes with repetition while it improves after the initial several contractions in the latter. In addition, patients may present with ptosis that is worse at the end of the day. The ptosis is typically not present in the morning.

A. Lambert Eaton → Incorrect. Lambert Eaton improves with use and symptoms will be worst in the morning. Strength will improve with repetitive motion. It is also a paraneoplastic syndrome associated with small cell lung cancers.

C. Narcolepsy → Incorrect. Although the patient has a complaint of "fatigue," she never mentions difficulty with sleep, so disorders such as narcolepsy are less likely.

D. Multiple sclerosis → Incorrect. Unlikely, as there is no evidence of lesions disseminated in space and time.

E. Parkinson disease → Incorrect. Does not exhibit the tetrad of parkinsonian symptoms: bradykinesia, rigidity, resting tremor, and shuffling gait

2. WWGJD? A 60-year-old man comes to the physician with muscle weakness and cramping that has been ongoing for the past 4 months. On exam, the patient was found to have **hyperactive deep tendon reflexes, fasiculations and muscle atrophy** in the left and right leg as well as right wrist drop. There were no abnormalities in the sensory or proprioceptive examinations. Given his clinical presentation, **what diagnosis does the patient most likely have?**

Answer: D, Amyotrophic lateral sclerosis

Explanation: This patient has both upper (hyperactive reflexes) and lower motor neuron (fasciculations and atrophy) signs. Combined with the distal > proximal weakness makes ALS the most likely diagnosis, as it is the only choice that would affect both upper and lower motor neurons.

A. Guillain-Barre syndrome → Incorrect. Presents with lower motor neuron damage.

B. Cauda equina → Incorrect. This condition leads to severe radicular pain and sensory and motor deficits due to compression of the cauda equine.

C. Multipole sclerosis → Incorrect. MS presents with upper motor signs only.

E. Myasthenia gravis → Incorrect. We are not given a history of fluctuating weakness, and the pattern of distal > proximal limb weakness is not a good fit for myasthenia gravis.

3. WWGJD? A 55-year-old female presents to a dermatologist with a violet rash around her eyes and red papules over the joints of her fingers. She notes that she's been feeling tired lately and has been having trouble stocking the highest shelves while volunteering at the food pantry. She thinks she has lost weight recently and hasn't seen her primary care doctor for several years. When the appointment is over the dermatologist has to help her out of her chair. Which of the following answer choices is correct?

Answer: B, A mammography should be ordered

Explanation: The patient in this question has dermatomyositis. She presents with proximal weakness (unable to lift things overhead and can't rise out of chair) with the distinctive heliotrope rash and Gottron papules. She also has been losing weight and has not been receiving appropriate cancer screening for several years. Dermatomyositis and polymyositis are associated with carcinomas, so an appropriate course of action would be to screen for common malignancies, such as breast cancer in this case.

A. Corticosteroids would not be expected to improve the weakness → Incorrect. This is true for inclusion body myositis. Dermatomyositis, however, does respond to steroids.

C. Neostigmine would lead to increased strength → Incorrect. This is true of myasthenia gravis.

D. A muscle biopsy would show CD8+ T cells in the endomysium → Incorrect. These are the findings of polymyositis. Dermatomyositis would show perimysial B cells with perifascicular atrophy.

Notes

Movement Disorders

Michael Baer, Leo Wang, Hao-Hua Wu, and Chuang-Kuo Wu

Movement Disorders

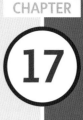

Movement disorders refer to diseases that result in either too much movement (hyperkinetic) or too little movement (hypokinetic). They factor prominently into the shelf exam, with the heaviest focus on Parkinson disease (PD). To provide a framework for study, the disorders will be grouped as hypokinetic or hyperkinetic. The only hypokinetic disorder that will be discussed is PD, a common neurodegenerative condition characterized by bradykinesia, rigidity, resting tremor, and postural instability. The hyperkinetic disorders include Huntington disease (HD), essential tremor (ET), acute dystonia, and Tourette syndrome. While studying this chapter, focus on the key movements in the presentation of each disease (Table 17.1) It is important to note that the distinction between hypokinetic and hyperkinetic disorders is not perfect (i.e., both ET and PD are both characterized by tremor), but it refers to the overall clinical picture. Finally, many movement disorders, such as tardive dyskinesia, are caused by medication side effects and are discussed in Chapter 11.

While the pathophysiology of movement disorders is extremely complex, with derangements in multiple basal ganglia and thalamic pathways, most shelf questions can be answered without complete memorization of these circuits. Therefore, a brief introduction to the neural pathways of movement will be provided. It may also be helpful to review preclinical material if the concepts seem confusing. This will give context to the actions of therapies and the pathologies of the disease presented.

The Neuroanatomy of Movement Disorders

The main player when it comes to movement disorders is the basal ganglia, a collection of different nuclei connected through several circuits. It includes the caudate and putamen (together called the striatum), the globus pallidus, the subthalamic nucleus, and the substantia nigra. Running within the basal ganglia are two pathways: the direct pathway and the

TABLE 17.1 Common Movement Disorder Terms

Movement	Description	Association
Resting tremor	Suppressed by activity	Parkinson
Action tremor	Increased during motor activity	Essential tremor
Intention tremor	Present at end of purposeful movement	Cerebellar lesions
Chorea	Involuntary wild jerking movements	Huntington
Dystonia	Sustained contractions causing abnormal posture/repetitive movements	Acute dystonic reactions
Tic	Sudden, involuntary, stereotyped motor movements or vocalizations preceded by urge	Tourette

indirect pathway. Put simply, activation of the direct pathway allows the motor cortex to initiate movement, and activation of the indirect pathway prevents movement. Activation of the direct pathway and inactivation of the indirect pathway can be achieved with dopamine from the substantia nigra, which connects with neurons in the striatum (caudate and putamen). We can now explain two important disorders. In PD, diseased cells in the substantia nigra are destroyed, so less dopamine is released. This means that the direct pathway is less activated, and the indirect pathway is less inactivated (or more activated!). The balance is tipped towards the indirect pathway and movement becomes difficult to initiate. In HD, the indirect pathway neurons in the striatum are damaged. This leads to an imbalance in favor of the direct pathway and wild, jerky movements.

gg AR

Direct and indirect pathways

gg AR

The direct and indirect pathways in Parkinson and Huntington

Hypokinetic Disorders

A. Parkinson Disease

Buzz Words: Cogwheel rigidity + resting tremor + shuffling gait + bradykinesia + postural instability + micrographia + respond to levodopa + dementia after 12 months

Clinical Presentation: PD is the second most common neurodegenerative disease (after Alzheimer) and is caused by the deposition of alpha-synuclein in the pigmented nuclei of the brainstem. The shelf exam tests your ability to recognize the diagnostic features of PD and the available therapies. In addition, PD patients sometimes develop dementia, and some patients with PD symptoms develop dementia very early in their disease course. These patients will have more widespread alpha-synuclein deposition and diagnosed with Lewy body dementia. Parkinson can also be considered a **hypo**kinetic movement disorder.

The chief complaint will likely be one of four complaints: bradykinesia, resting tremor, postural instability, cogwheel rigidity. There is a possible link to repeated head trauma and organophosphate exposure may increase risk (toxic to dopaminergic substantia nigra neurons).

PPx: None

MoD: Lewy bodies (alpha-synuclein aggregates) accumulate in brainstem pigmented nuclei (including substantia nigra) → Leads to neuronal death and loss of dopaminergic neurons in substantia nigra

- The bradykinesia is secondary to loss of dopaminergic neurons in the substantia nigra. The direct pathway receives less activation (so indirect > direct) → movement difficult to initiate

Dx:

1. Clinical exam with resting "pill rolling" tremor, bradykinesia, rigidity.
2. Magnetic resonance imaging/computed tomography (MRI/CT to rule out mimics of PD.
3. Favorable response with levodopa
4. DaTSCAN (SPECT scan using dopamine transporter labeled tracer; detection of dopamine uptake deficiency in caudate and putamen)
   - **Normal pressure hydrocephalus** may mimic the gait and postural instability of Parkinson and can be treated with an LP.
   - **ET** may be confused with PD, but the ET tremor is made worse with **action**, and the PD tremor is worse at **rest.**
   - **Progressive supranuclear** palsy (PSP) may present with rigidity and falls (instability) but has a vertical gaze palsy.
   - Parkinson symptoms and dementia occurring at roughly the same time should bring up Lewy body dementia.

Tx/Mgmt:

1. Treatment cannot reverse the alpha-synuclein pathology, but focuses on symptom management.
   - Levodopa-carbidopa → replaces dopamine lost with damage of substantia nigra
     - Carbidopa is a decarboxylase inhibitor (prevents degradation of levodopa before it gets to the brain)

QUICK TIPS
Postural instability = loss of reflexes that maintain posture (leads to falls)

- COMT inhibitors are also used with levodopa to extent plasma half-life (COMT degrades levodopa)
  - Main side effect is dyskinesias → involuntary jerking movements
- MAO-B inhibitors (rasagiline, selegiline) may improve motor symptoms alone or complement the effects of levodopa
  - MAO-B breaks down dopamine in the CNS
- Dopamine agonists (bromocriptine, pramipexole) → direct effect of effect on striatal neurons, less potent than levodopa
  - Main side effects are hypotension and hallucinations/confusion
- Anticholinergic agents (benztropine) → tremor reduction, less impact on bradykinesia
- Deep Brain Stimulation if medication fails
  - Electrodes inhibit subthalamic nucleus (indirect pathway)

99 AR

Mechanisms of Parkinson's therapies

Hyperkinetic Disorders

B. Huntington Disease

Buzz Words: Atrophy of the caudate nucleus + forgetfulness + family history of early death + change in personality + chorea + depression

Clinical Presentation: HD is an autosomal dominant condition caused by CAG repeat expansions in the *huntingtin* gene. Patients exhibit wild jerking movements (chorea) and dementia as prominent features. Many patients develop depression, and the suicide rate is quite high. No effective therapies exist. Patients typically first report personality changes (depression, impulsivity, irritability), diminished attention/concentration with preserved memory, patient appears "fidgety" with later development of widespread chorea. Family history of chorea/early death, disease manifests at younger age with each generation (anticipation, see later for explanation).

99 AR

Choreiform movements

PPx:

1. Genetic testing/counseling

MoD: CAG repeats in Huntington gene on chromosome 4 expand during replication → increasing lengths = more severe/younger onset of disease → CAG expansion = expansion of polyglutamine region of huntingtin protein → proteins aggregate in neuron nuclei → loss of GABA and ACh containing neurons in basal ganglia → atrophy of caudate and putamen

- The mutant huntingtin protein may also interrupt

transcriptional proteins or sensitize cells to glutamate excitotoxicity

- Chorea results from destruction of striatal neurons
(caudate + putamen) in the indirect pathway (less
indirect pathway = more movement)
- Anticipation = earlier onset in successive generations.
During meiosis, the CAG repeats can expand so children may have longer expansions than the parents

Dx:

1. Family history with genetic testing for CAG repeats
(>39) (2)CT/MRI with atrophy of caudate/putamen and
enlarged ventricles

Tx/Mgmt: Treatment focuses on controlling the chorea by
decreasing effect of dopamine

Caudate atrophy in HD

- Haloperidol (dopamine antagonist)
- Tetrabenazine/reserpine (decrease dopamine re-
lease as VMAT inhibitors)
- Antidepressants for depression/suicidality

C. Essential Tremor

Buzz Words: Symmetrical action tremor of the hands +
quivering of the voice (vocal tremor) + difficulty with
precise tasks (threading needle) + better with alcohol/
propranolol

Clinical Presentation: ET (benign tremor or familial tremor) is
the most common type of tremor. It commonly affects
the arms and is worsened with movement (action tremor).
Alcohol diminishes the tremor and anxiety, exercise,
and fatigue make it worse. The tremor is often familial,
exhibiting an autosomal dominant inheritance pattern.
ET should be distinguished from an intention tremor,
which is caused by cerebellar dysfunction and presents when reaching for an object. Intention tremors
are seen in patients with multiple sclerosis, Wilson
disease, and cerebrovascular disease. ET is also
confused with PD, so be sure to learn the difference
between an action tremor and a resting tremor.

PPx: None

MoD: Unknown, and no genes have been identified in
familial cases

Dx:

1. Clinical exam with symmetrical (usually) action tremor

Tx/Mgmt:

1. Propranolol (beta agonist activity)
2. Primidone (barbiturate)
3. Gabapentin, topiramate, mirtazapine for refractory
cases

D. Acute Dystonia

Buzz Words: Abnormal posturing/position + worse with movement + neuroleptic exposure

Clinical Presentation: Acute dystonia does not refer to a single clinical entity, but is instead a product of a variety of underlying causes. Dystonias are involuntary muscle contractions resulting in abnormal postures and movements and can be limited to one part of the body, one side of the body, or most/all of the body (generalized). The list of underlying causes is large and includes neonatal hypoxia, kernicterus, AIDs, lysosomal storage disorders, and neurodegenerative diseases like HD, PSP, and PD. The most commonly encountered dystonias are those restricted to parts of the body like the neck (torticollis), orbicularis oculi (blepharospasm), and hand (writer's cramp). Another important category is the dystonia caused by neuroleptics.

PPx: None

MoD: Variable due to multiple underlying pathologies. Neuroleptic induced dystonia is likely caused by antagonism of the D2 receptor. Haloperidol, fluphenazine, and metoclopramide are commonly associated with dystonias.

Dx:

1. Clinical exam with repetitive, unnatural spasmodic movements (neuroleptic associated dystonia most commonly involves muscles around mouth, the tongue, or the neck)

Tx/Mgmt:

1. For neuroleptic associated dystonia, stop offending agent and try diphenhydramine or benztropine

E. Tourette Syndrome

Buzz Words: repetitive sniffing/snorting/vocalization + compulsive behavior + ADHD

Clinical Presentation: Tics are sudden, involuntary, stereotyped motor movements, or vocalizations that are accompanied by an irresistible urge relieved by movement. Tourette is the most severe tic syndrome and is characterized by multiple motor and vocal tics. The disorder begins in childhood, has a male predominance, and is associated with ADHD and obsessive compulsive behavior. Like Sydenham chorea, a portion of Tourette cases are related to streptococcal infection (PANDAS—pediatric autoimmune neuropsychiatric disorders with streptococcal infection).

99 AR

Side effects of antipsychotics

PPx: None

MoD: Unknown, may involve abnormalities of dopamine signaling in the caudate (levodopa makes Sx worse, haloperidol makes Sx better)

Dx:
1. Multiple motor and vocal tics
2. Tics occur many times/day
3. Onset before 21
4. Location, number, type, severity of tics change over time
5. Not explained by medication/substance/medical condition
   - In ½ of adolescents, the tics subside before adulthood

Tx/Mgmt:
1. Alpha2 adrenergic agonists (clonidine and guanfacine)
2. Antipsychotics (haloperidol, pimozide, risperidone)
3. Hyperactivity treated with methylphenidate or clonidine (Table 17.2)

TABLE 17.2 Summary of Movement Disorders

Disease	Abnormal movement	MoA	Treatment
Parkinson	Resting tremor + bradykinesia + shuffling gait	Loss of dopaminergic substantia nigra	Replace dopamine (levodopa-carbidopa)
Essential Tremor	Action tremor	Unknown	Beta2 adrenergic blockade (propranolol)
Huntington	Chorea	CAG expansion of *huntington* → damage of caudate/putamen	Decrease dopamine (Haloperidol)
Acute dystonia (antipsychotic related)	Involuntary contractions—abnormal postures	D2 receptor antagonism	Diphenhydramine or benztropine
Tourette	Multiple tics	Unknown	Alpha2 adrenergic agonists (clonidine or guanfacine)

GUNNER PRACTICE

1. A 63-year-old male presents to a neurologist with a tremor of his hands. He says he notices the tremor when reaching out to turn off a light or ring a doorbell. An avid drinker, he doesn't think the tremor is better or worse with alcohol. He was admitted to the hospital twice in the last 5 years for strokes. An examination reveals a tremor that worsens during the finger to nose test. Which of the following is the correct answer choice?
   A. Other family members likely have the same tremor.
   B. The tremor should respond well to propranolol.
   C. A brain MRI may show a remote cerebellar infarct.
   D. A lumbar puncture should be performed for symptomatic relief.

2. An 11-year-old boy is brought into the clinic by his parents because of uncontrollable movements of his entire body. These movements have been increasing in frequency and intensity. He has no history of seizures, loss of consciousness, or head trauma. His mom mentions that he had a sore throat a month ago. There is no significant family history, although the patient's paternal grandfather has dementia. His blood pressure is 90/50, respirations are 12/min, pulse is 95/min, and temperature is 98.7°F. On examination, spasmodic jerking movements are appreciated in the upper and lower extremities. The remainder of the examination shows no abnormalities. Neuroimaging and an electroencephalogram (EEG) show no abnormalities. Which of the following is the most likely diagnosis?
   A. Early-onset HD
   B. General tonic seizures
   C. Sydenham chorea
   D. Tourette disorder

3. A 45-year-old female presents to her doctor accompanied by her husband. He says that she has become increasingly irritable over the past year, which is entirely out of character for her. Some of her work colleagues have volunteered that her high level of concentration has diminished and she appears nervous and fidgety, and her work performance as an accountant has begun to slip. Her father committed suicide in his early 50s, and her grandfather passed away from dementia. On examination, the patient appears markedly restless and

is unable to keep her arms or legs still. Which of the following is false?

A. The patient should be carefully screened for depression.
B. Levodopa will improve her restlessness.
C. Her symptoms result from aggregation of abnormal proteins in the striatum.
D. Her children may show similar symptoms before the age of 45.

ANSWERS: What Would Gunner Jess/Jim Do?

1. WWGJD? A 63-year-old male presents to a neurologist with a tremor of his right hand. He says he notices the tremor when reaching out to turn off a light or ring a doorbell. An avid drinker, he doesn't think the tremor is better or worse with alcohol. He was admitted to the hospital twice in the last five years for strokes. An examination reveals a tremor that worsens during the finger to nose test. Which of the following is the correct answer choice?

Answer: C, A brain MRI may show a remote cerebellar infarct

Explanation: This patient presents with an intention tremor, which occurs at the end of a purposeful movement, like ringing a doorbell. These are associated with lesions in the cerebellum that can be caused by stroke, alcoholism, and multiple sclerosis. Given our patient's history of stroke, the best answer from the choices above is that his intention tremor is caused by a remote infarct to the cerebellum.

A. Other family members likely have the same tremor → Incorrect. This is true for ET, which often has a familial component.

B. The tremor should respond well to propranolol → Incorrect. ET responds best to propranolol.

D. A lumbar puncture should be performed for symptomatic relief → Incorrect. This is true of normal pressure hydrocephalus, which presents with the triad of dementia, urinary incontinence, and wobbly gait.

2. WWGJD? An 11-year-old boy is brought into the clinic by his parents because of uncontrollable movements of his entire body. These movements have been increasing in frequency and intensity. He has no history of seizures, loss of consciousness or head trauma. His mom mentions that he had a sore throat a month ago. There is no significant family history, although the patient's paternal grandfather has dementia. Her blood pressure is 90/50, respirations are 12/min, pulse is 95/min, and temperature is 98.7F. On examination, spasmodic jerking movements are appreciated in the upper and lower extremities. The remainder of the examination shows no abnormalities. Neuroimaging and an EEG show no abnormalities. Which of the following is the most likely diagnosis?

Answer: C, Sydenham chorea

Explanation: Given the patient's history of a sore throat and normal CT and EEG, it is likely that he has Sydenham chorea secondary to acute rheumatic fever. The movements, described as jerking, spasmodic, and uncontrollable, appear choreiform.

A. Early onset HD → Incorrect. This is less likely, given the lack of family history of dementia with chorea.

B. General tonic seizures → Incorrect. In a generalized seizure, the patient would not be alert and oriented, eliminating this diagnosis.

D. Tourette Disorder → Incorrect. While Tourette syndrome can present acutely following a strep infection, the movements described in the question (jerking, spasmodic) fit more with a chorea. In addition, the patient does not note an urge preceding the actions, which would fit a tic disorder.

3. WWGJD? A 45-year-old female presents to her doctor accompanied by her husband. He says that she has become increasingly irritable over the past year, which is entirely out of character for her. Some of her work colleagues have volunteered that her high level of concentration has diminished and she appears nervous and fidgety, and her work performance as an accountant has begun to slip. Her father committed suicide in his early 50s and her grandfather passed away from dementia. On examination the patient appears markedly restless and is unable to keep her arms or legs still. Which of the following is false?

Answer: B, Levodopa will improve her restlessness.

Explanation: The question stem describes HD. The patient is exhibiting personality and cognitive changes, which are commonly seen in HD. She also is markedly restless, and can't hold her arms and legs still, consistent with the early abnormal movements of HD. Her father committed suicide (common in HD) and her grandfather had dementia (end result of HD). Levodopa will worsen her movement disorder, while dopamine antagonists would improve it.

A. The patient should be carefully screened for depression → Incorrect. This is true, as HD has a high depression/suicide rate.

C. Her symptoms result from aggregation of abnormal proteins in the striatum → Incorrect. The CAG repeat expansions in the *huntingtin* gene lead to an abnormal huntingtin protein which can aggregate in neuronal nuclei, notably the caudate and putamen (striatum).

D. Her children may show similar symptoms before the age of 45 → Incorrect. HD is passed along as an autosomal dominant and exhibits anticipation, with children exhibiting symptoms at a younger age than the parents. During gametogenesis, the CAG repeats can increase in number and the number of repeats are associated with age of onset and severity of the disease.

Congenital Disorders of the Neurology Shelf

Hao-Hua Wu, Leo Wang, and Chuang-Kuo Wu

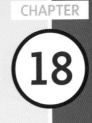

All of the disorders mentioned in this chapter can be tested on either the neuro or pediatric shelf. Although there are some details included that probably do not need to be known for the neuro shelf (such as the mechanism of disease for these congenital disorders), it is good to familiarize yourself with these diseases. Since congenital disorders are often not treatable, the National Board of Medical Examiners (NBME) can only test you on buzz words and leave it to you to diagnose the disease. Thus, memorize the buzz words for popular test topics, like fetal alcohol syndrome (FAS) and Down syndrome, and you will do well on exam day.

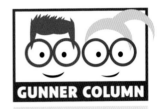

GUNNER COLUMN

Congenital Disorders

A. Friedreich Ataxia

Buzz Words: <22 years (onset during teenage years) + gait ataxia + frequent falling + dysarthria + hypertrophic cardiomyopathy + diabetes + hammer toes + pes cavus + scoliosis + loss of position/vibration + pain/temp still intact

Clinical Presentation: Friedreich ataxia is the most common type of autosomal recessive spinocerebellar ataxia. Most common cause of death of patients with Friedreich ataxia (mean survival 20 years from diagnosis) is cardiomyopathy. Respiratory is the second most common. Pes cavus can also be Charcot-Marie-Tooth disease, so make sure to differentiate accordingly.

PPx: Genetic consultation for future pregnancies

MoD: AR disorder that begins <22 years on chromosome 9, GAA repeat → disorder of frataxin, an iron binding protein → damage of posterior columns
- Frataxin is needed for mitochondrial iron regulation → loss of regulation leads to iron build up/free radical damage

Dx:
1. Clinical Exam
2. Southern Blot
3. Echo to look for HCM

Tx/Mgmt:
1. Supportive
2. Treatment of HCM

B. Neural Tube Defects (NTDs)

Just know the definitions and ways to prevent (as most NTDs result in congenital deaths), most commonly folate intake

1. Spina bifida = failure of posterior vertebral arch to close
   a. can ppx with maternal folate supplementation
   b. Meningocele = protrusion of meninges in spina bifida
   c. Meningomyelocele = protrusion of meninges and spinal cord in spina bifida
2. Holoprosencephaly = forebrain fails to develop into two hemispheres → death
3. Anencephaly = failure of cranial end of neural tube to form → absence of skull/brain → death

C. Sturge-Weber Syndrome

Buzz Words: Port wine stain aka nevus flammeus + congenital unilateral cavernous hemangioma along trigeminal nerve distribution + intracranial calcifications that resemble a tramline + generalized seizures + mental retardation

Clinical Presentation: Sturge-Weber Syndrome is a genetic disorder caused by a GNAQ gene mutation that is characterized by the port wine stain on the neurology shelf. It is NOT THE SAME as tuberous sclerosis (infantile spasms = tuberous sclerosis = associated with adenoma sebaceum). Unlike tuberous sclerosis, patients with Sturge-Weber suffer from generalized seizures. The most common complications of this disorder are hemisensory disturbance, ipsilateral glaucoma, and hemianopia.

PPx: None

MoD: GNAQ gene mutation

Dx:
1. Computed tomography (CT) to r/o tumors
2. Electroencephalogram (EEG) to monitor seizures

Tx/Mgmt:
1. Argon laser therapy to remove skin lesions and reduce intraocular pressure
2. Levetiracetam (Keppra) for generalized seizures

D. Tuberous Sclerosis (Tuberous Sclerosis Complex—TSC)

Buzz words: Hypopigmented macules (ash leaf spots) (Fig. 18.1) + facial angiofibromas (Fig. 18.2) + cardiac rhabdomyomas + renal angioleiomyomas + MR + seizures + astrocytoma + infantile spasms

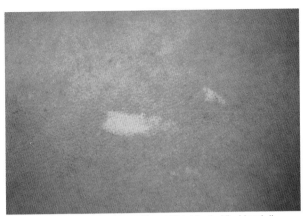

FIG. 18.1 Ash leaf spots. (From Siegel DH, Martin KL, Hand JL. Selected hereditary diseases. In: Eichenfield LF, Frieden IJ, Mathes EF, et al., eds. *Neonatal and Infant Dermatology*. 3rd ed. London: Saunders; 2014.)

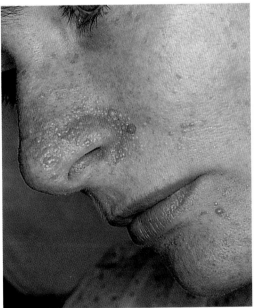

FIG. 18.2 Angiofibromas. (From Gawkrodger DJ, Ardem-Jones MR. Neurocutaneous disorders and other syndromes. In: Gawkrodger DJ, Ardern-Jones MR, eds. *Dermatology: An Illustrated Colour Text*, 5th ed. London: Elsevier Ltd., 2012.)

Clinical Presentation: Tuberous sclerosis is a genetic disorder characterized by TSC1/2 mutations. It is most easily identified in a question stem by ash leaf spots and infantile spasms. Make sure to differentiate from Sturge-Weber, which instead presents with generalized seizures.

PPx: None

MoD: TSC1 and TSC2 gene mutations (TSC1—Chromosome 9—hamartin; TSC2—Chromosome 16—tuberin) → impaired the mTOR (mammalian target of rapamycin) pathway → tuberous sclerosis

Dx:

1. Look for ash leaf spots and angiofibromas
2. EEG
3. Magnetic resonance imaging (MRI) to r/o structural etiology
4. Pyruvate, lactate, amino acids, to r/o metabolism disorders
5. Consult optho to r/o TORCH infection
6. Genome wide sequencing to look for mutations like STXBP1, CASK and PNPO
7. CXR to rule out TB (since that is contraindication for ACTH therapy)

Tx/Mgmt:

1. Anticipatory guidance for parents
2. Treatment of infantile spasms (Tx with ACTH)

E. von Hippel-Lindau (VHL) Disease

Buzz Words: Bilateral renal cell carcinoma (RCC) + hemangioblastoma + pheochromocytoma + retinal angioma

Clinical Presentation: von Hippel-Lindau disease is most commonly associated with hemangioblastoma on the shelf. Do not get confused with tuberous sclerosis, which is associated with hamartomas and not hemangioblastomas.

PPx: None

MoD: Autosomal dominant mutation of VHL gene, chromosome 3

- RCC occurs because VHL gene is a tumor suppressor gene

Dx:

1. Measurement of catecholamines in blood
2. Metanephrines in the urine

Tx/Mgmt:

1. Surgical resection of adrenal gland tumor
2. Antihypertensives
3. Treatment of RCC

F. Down Syndrome

Buzz Words:

- Simian crease, big tongue, white spots on iris, decreased tone, oblique palpebral fissures, epicanthal folds → Down syndrome

- Hypothyroidism + Hirschsprung + duodenal atresia + complete AV canal defect + **early-onset Alzheimer**→ Down syndrome
  - Failure of endocardial cushion fusion results in AV septal defects
  - Complete AV septal defects causes heart failure in early infancy and requires surgical repair
- Hyperreflexia in legs + urinary incontinence + hypotonic + b/l Babinski reflex + in s/o Down syndrome → atlantoaxial instability → 2/2 atlantoaxial instability of C1/C2 in down syndrome

Clinical Presentation: Down syndrome is the most commonly tested subject in this chapter. It appears multiple times in the neurology shelf and is likely to appear on all other shelf exams you take. Pay close attention to the Buzz Words of babies born with Down syndrome (e.g., simian crease, epicanthal fold) and be sure to memorize high-yield complications, such as early-onset Alzheimer and hypothyroidism.

PPx:
1. Bear child at younger age (<35 years)

MoD: Trisomy 21

Dx:
1. Lateral radiographs of cervical spine in flexion + open mouth radiographs to visualize odontoid to r/o atlantoaxial instability

Tx/Mgmt: Treat based on complications (e.g., If atlantoaxial instability → fusion of C1 and C2)

G. Fetal Alcohol Syndrome

Buzz Words: Midfacial hypoplasia + microcephaly + stunted growth + mental retardation but no cleft palate or excess hair (Fig. 18.3) → FAS

Smooth philtrum (Fig. 18.4) + thin vermillion border + small palpebral fissures (horizontal space between lateral and medial canthal fold) → FAS

Complications of FAS include: Fetal alcohol dysmorphism + social withdrawal + delays in motor/language milestones + ADHD → complications of FAS

Clinical Presentation: FAS is a commonly tested subject and is most easily identified by a patient's "smooth philtrum" or "missing philtrum."

PPx: Mom avoids alcohol. (No safe amount of prenatal alcohol consumption!)

MoD: Unknown

Dx:
1. Clinical exam

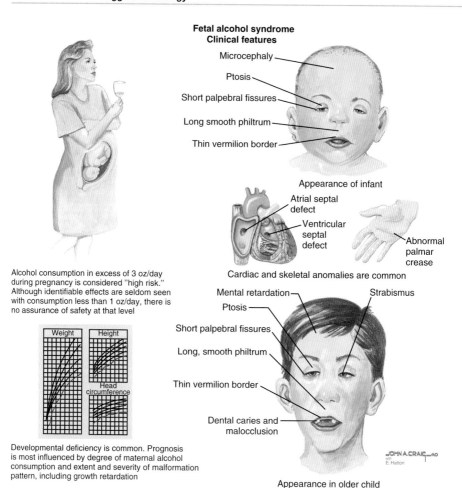

Fetal alcohol syndrome
Clinical features

Microcephaly

Ptosis

Short palpebral fissures

Long smooth philtrum

Thin vermilion border

Appearance of infant

Atrial septal defect

Ventricular septal defect

Abnormal palmar crease

Alcohol consumption in excess of 3 oz/day during pregnancy is considered "high risk." Although identifiable effects are seldom seen with consumption less than 1 oz/day, there is no assurance of safety at that level

Cardiac and skeletal anomalies are common

Mental retardation   Strabismus

Ptosis

Short palpebral fissures

Long, smooth philtrum

Thin vermilion border

Dental caries and malocclusion

Weight   Height

Head circumference

Developmental deficiency is common. Prognosis is most influenced by degree of maternal alcohol consumption and extent and severity of malformation pattern, including growth retardation

Appearance in older child

FIG. 18.3 Fetal alcohol syndrome facies. (Copyright 2016 Elsevier Inc. All rights reserved. www.netterim ages.com.)

Tx/Mgmt:

1. Supportive care
2. Learning support for child growing up

H. Rett's Disorder (5 Months)

Buzz Words: Female + decreased head circumference growth rate during 5–48 months + loss of previously acquired hand skills after 5 months + severely impaired language + severely impaired psychomotor development + stereotyped hand movements + trunk/gait problem + cyanotic spells + seizures

Clinical Presentation: Rett disorder is caused by an abnormality on the X-chromosome and is associated with MECP-2 gene. It is a disease that only girls can get. The most common findings include small head, hands, feet, and repetitive hand movements. Rett's was recently

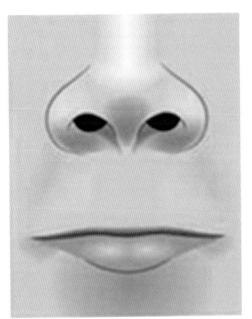

FIG. 18.4 Smooth philtrum of infant born with fetal alcohol syndrome. (From Mukherjee RAS. Fetal alcohol spectrum disorders. *Paediatr Child Health*. 2015;25(12):580–586.)

removed from the DSM and is more often categorized as a neurologic disorder. Of note, the previous name of Rett's syndrome, cerebroatrophic hyperammonemia, has nothing to do with the disease itself and high ammonia levels were an incidental finding. Be sure to rule out childhood disintegrative disorder, in which the patient will only start deteriorating after 2 years of age.

PPx: Screen females who were normal for first 5 months of life and started deteriorating

MoA: Associated with MECP2 gene on X-chromosome

Dx:

1. Vision and hearing test to r/o medical cause
2. Lab tests for lead
3. Genetic test (chromosomal analyses)

Tx/Mgmt:

1. Speech and language eval
2. Psychological supportive treatment counseling for patient and family

GUNNER PRACTICE

1. A 6-month-old boy is brought to the physician because of a 1-week history of episodes of unprovoked startle-like movements. Each movement consists of sudden, quick flexion of the head, arms, and legs. He cries during

these movements, which usually occur in clusters after awakening from sleep. He has had a heart murmur since birth. His father has mild mental impairment. Examination shows three areas of skin hypopigmentation, each measuring 1–2 cm. A CT scan of the head shows four periventricular nodules that distort the normally smooth ventricular margins. Which of the following is the most likely diagnosis?

A. Duchenne muscular dystrophy
B. Facioscapulohumeral muscular dystrophy
C. Hepatolenticular degeneration (Wilson disease)
D. Myotonic dystrophy
E. Neurofibromatosis
F. Tuberous sclerosis

2. An 18-year-old man comes to his physician for a routine maintenance examination. Since he was 3, he has been unable to relax his hands after tightly gripping objects or after shaking hands. His family history is notable for cataracts and frontal baldness in his father. Physical examination shows atrophy in his lower arms, and there is moderate weakness of his hands with difficulty releasing grip after flexion. Which of the following is the most likely diagnosis?

A. Polymyalgia rheumatica
B. Polymyositis
C. Cervical spondylosis
D. Amyotrophic lateral sclerosis
E. Myasthenic (Lambert-Eaton) syndrome
F. Myotonic muscular dystrophy
G. Multiple sclerosis
H. Myasthenia gravis

3. An 11-year-old boy is brought to his physician due to a 6-month-history of difficulty walking and leg pain. Physical examination shows atrophy in his legs with hammer toes. Which diagnostic procedure would be most relevant in managing the most common cause of death in this patient?

A. Echocardiogram
B. EEG
C. Gower maneuver
D. Electromyography (EMG)
E. Muscle biopsy

Notes

ANSWERS: What Would Gunner Jess/Jim Do?

1. WWGJD? A 6-month-old boy is brought to the physician because of a 1-week history of episodes of unprovoked startle-like movements. Each movement consists of sudden, quick flexion of the head, arms, and legs. He cries during these movements, which usually occur in clusters after awakening from sleep. He has had a heart murmur since birth. His father has mild mental impairment. Examination shows three areas of skin hypopigmentation, each measuring 12 cm. A CT scan of the head shows four periventricular nodules that distort the normally smooth ventricular margins. Which of the following is the most likely diagnosis?

Answer: F, Tuberous sclerosis

Explanation: This is a boy that is showing signs of infantile spasm (i.e., "sudden, quick flexion of head, arms, and legs"). Also, giving it away are the shagreen patches seen with "three areas of skin hypopigmentation," another classic buzz word for tuberous sclerosis. None of the other answer choices lead to infantile spasm-like movements and can all be ruled out.

A. Duchenne muscular dystrophy (DMD) → Incorrect. DMD is a defect in dystrophin that leads to muscle weakness. It does not manifest as any type of spasming by a 6-month-old child.

B. Facioscapulohumeral muscular dystrophy → Incorrect. Facioscapulohumeral muscular dystrophy is a rare disease that only affects the muscles of the face, scapula, and humerus (which one can ascertain from the name). Since this patient does not have face, scapular, or humeral muscle involvement, this answer choice can be ruled out.

C. Hepatolenticular degeneration (Wilson disease) → Incorrect. Wilson disease is not associated with tumors of the ventricle or skin hypopigmentation. Thus, C can be ruled out.

D. Myotonic dystrophy → Incorrect. Myotonic dystrophy is a chronic, slowly progressing form of muscular dystrophy. Since this patient is only 6 months old, it is unlikely he will show symptoms of myotonic dystrophy.

E. Neurofibromatosis → Incorrect. Although NF1 or NF2 can present with intracranial tumors, it does not lead to infantile spasms or shagreen spots. Instead, the cutaneous manifestation would be café au lait spots.

2. WWGJD? An 18-year-old man comes to his physician for a routine maintenance examination. Since he was three, he has been unable to relax his hands after tightly gripping objects or after shaking hands. His family history is notable for cataracts and frontal baldness in his father. Physical examination shows atrophy in his lower arms, and there is moderate weakness of his hands with difficulty releasing grip after flexion. Which of the following is the most likely diagnosis?

Answer: F, Myotonic muscular dystrophy

Explanation: This is the second most common muscular dystrophy in America. Both skeletal muscle and smooth muscle are affected, and patients have other problems including immunologic deficiencies, cardiac arrhythmias, cataracts, and frontal balding (due to hormonal abnormalities). Inability to release grip (especially from doorknobs) is typical for this disease process. Look for this pattern to be passed from generation to generation.

A. Polymyalgia rheumatica → Incorrect. This syndrome involves pain and stiffness in large joints like the neck, shoulder, upper arms, and hips and is coincident with temporal arteritis. Notably, there is no weakness. This patient exhibits weakness but no pain, making polymyalgia rheumatica incorrect.

B. Polymyositis → Incorrect. The hallmark of polymyositis is weakness and pain in proximal musculature, especially in the hip flexors. This patient does not exhibit pain and the weakness is only present during hand grip. Moreover, polymyositis is more prevalent in females and is not passed from generation to generation.

C. Cervical spondylosis → Incorrect. This is typically caused by osteoarthritis, leading to cervical spine degeneration. Whereas this may lead to a radiculopathy causing these symptoms, it would be rare to see such a specific manifestation of it. There is also no inheritance pattern to cervical spondylosis, so the father having cataracts and frontal balding is unlikely.

D. Amyotrophic lateral sclerosis → Incorrect. ALS would not present at such an early age and would lead to loss of muscle tone in more than a single muscle group.

E. Myasthenic (Lambert-Eaton) syndrome (LES) → Incorrect. LES is typically associated with small cell lung cancers, which this patient has no evidence of having and is too young for. Moreover, LES causes neuromuscular weakness in multiple locations that improves with usage. If this patient had LES, their handgrip weakness should improve the more it is applied.

G. Multiple sclerosis → Incorrect. MS would have to cause multiple different defects that present both in space and time. Typically, ocular symptoms are common as well.

H. Myasthenia gravis → Incorrect. Myasthenia gravis is not inherited and presents with weakness that gets worse with usage, typically coincident with thymomas.

3. WWGJD? An 11-year-old boy is brought to his physician due to a 6-month-history of difficulty walking and leg pain. Physical examination shows atrophy in his legs with hammer toes. Which diagnostic procedure would be most relevant in managing the most common cause of death in this patient?

Answer: A, Echocardiogram

Explanation: Charcot-Marie-Tooth disease is characterized by progress motor and sensory loss, and is the most common inherited neurologic disorder. Hammer toes are pathognomonic for this disease process. The most common cause of death in CMT is cardiomyopathy, for which an echo may prove useful.

B. EEG → Incorrect. EEG is used for seizure disorders, for which CMT has no indication.

C. Gower maneuver → Incorrect. Gower maneuver is useful in diagnosing Duchenne and Becker muscular dystrophy.

D. EMG → Incorrect. EMG is useful in diagnosis of CMT but is not useful in diagnosing the most common cause of death.

E. Muscle biopsy → Incorrect. Since this disease is neurologic in nature, a nerve biopsy would prove more useful than a muscle biopsy.

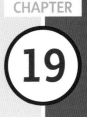
Gunner Jim's Guide to Exam Day Success

Hao-Hua Wu and Leo Wang

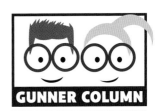

GUNNER COLUMN

Do these three things to perform well on any shelf:

1. Master one review book
2. Do as many quality questions as you can
3. Excel like a Gunner

"Master one review book"

Neurology clerkship rotations range from 2 to 4 weeks. That is not enough time to peruse multiple review books. The most important thing you can do prior to the start of your rotation is to identify the resource that best covers the material of the Neurology shelf. Once you have picked something, stick with it. The point of using a review book is so that you can get familiarized with the scope of the exam.

Most of your learning occurs when you complete questions, so don't be discouraged if you cannot memorize every word of your review book like you did for Step 1. Instead, use your review book as a point of reference and annotate the margins.

If you see one topic come up on multiple chapters (or maybe even multiple shelf exams), make sure to write down the page numbers where it appears and flip to those pages every time you review. The more connections you make between topics (e.g., thinking of Huntington disease as a disease process that can present as a movement disorder [chorea] and a degenerative disorder [dementia]) the more you will master.

In addition, highlight themes that keep coming up. For instance, anytime patients in the question recently change their medication regimen, suspect the medication change as the cause of their symptoms until proven otherwise. These organizing principles transcend individual topics and can help you do well on any shelf exam test question.

"Do as many quality questions as you can"

The key to success is practicing in an environment that simulates the pressure of test day, and nothing simulates that pressure better than taking practice questions under stringent time constraints.

After you identify your review book, select as many authoritative question banks as you can. We recommend Gunner Practice, UWorld, and NBME Clinical Science practice exams. Do at least 10 questions a day under timed conditions (1.5 minutes a question) starting on the first day of your rotation.

Remember, you can complete the same question multiple times in the course of study! In fact, it is recommended that you retry the questions you got wrong in the first place, just so that you know you will get it right on the test.

It is also important that the questions you complete are of high quality. This means that the length and content of the question stems reflect what you would actually see on test day. Many question bank resources are too easy (giving you a false sense of confidence) or ask about material that would not show up on the exam (wasting your time).

Once you have selected your question bank resources, count the total number of questions and divide it by the number of days you have available to study. Then make sure you set a study plan where you can make at least two passes through your questions. The first pass is completion of all available questions. The second pass is completion of all the questions you got wrong or made a lucky guess for during your first pass. Seeing how many of the second pass questions you get correct should be a nice confidence boost leading into exam day.

As you do questions, jot down patterns associated with the chief complaint. NBME question writers are instructed to write questions with a chief complaint that can plausibly be associated with at least five different diseases. Sharpen your differential after you read a question's first sentence and then use Buzz Words to narrow down your diagnosis. Once you reach your diagnosis, you will either be done with the question or have to draw upon knowledge of PPx, MoD, Dx, and Tx/Mgmt.

"Excel like a Gunner"

How you take notes for the questions you complete is imperative to success.

The most effective strategy is to pick **one** take home point for every question you complete and record it on an Excel sheet specific for your clinical rotation.

For instance, if you answer a question incorrectly about the treatment of absence seizures, write "Tx of absence seizures" in column A of your Excel sheet and then "Ethosuximide" in column B of your Excel sheet. This allows you to create an immediate, pseudo flashcard. When you review this material the following week, you can put your cursor over column A, say the answer out loud, and check your answer by shifting your cursor to column B. This saves time and emphasizes the most important takeaway for each question.

If you understand everything in the question and answer choices, don't record it in the Excel sheet.

If you don't understand multiple things in the question and answer choices, record the most important takeaway point and move on. For test day, it is better to be confident in what you know well than to undermine your confidence by fixating on what you are weak at.

By test day, you should have one excel sheet that contains one important take home point from every question you were unsure about. The tabs on the bottom should be organized by question bank resource. This Excel sheet would ideally only take 3–4 hours to review, and is something you would go over the day before the exam.

Last but not least, **trust the process.** Students often enter test day anxious and overwhelmed which can cause them to second-guess their answer choices. Trust the process—trust that you will have covered everything in leading up to the shelf exam and have some faith in your answer selections; for these reasons, don't second guess yourself. Your first instinct is usually right.

In summary: Read. Apply. Review. And prepare for success on test day!

Index

Note: Pages followed by "*b*", "*t*", and "*f*" refer to boxes, tables, and figures respectively.